WellMan

Live Longer by Controlling Inflammation

GRAHAM SIMPSON, M.D.

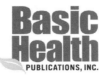

The information contained in this book is based upon the research and personal and professional experiences of the authors. It is not intended as a substitute for consulting with your physician or other healthcare provider. Any attempt to diagnose and treat an illness should be done under the direction of a healthcare professional.

The publisher does not advocate the use of any particular healthcare protocol but believes the information in this book should be available to the public. The publisher and authors are not responsible for any adverse effects or consequences resulting from the use of the suggestions, preparations, or procedures discussed in this book. Should the reader have any questions concerning the appropriateness of any procedures or preparation mentioned, the authors and the publisher strongly suggest consulting a professional healthcare advisor.

Basic Health Publications, Inc.
28812 Top of the World Drive
Laguna Beach, CA 92651
949-715-7327 • www.basichealthpub.com

Library of Congress Cataloging-in-Publication Data

Simpson, Graham
    Wellman : live longer by controlling inflammation / Graham Simpson.
      p. cm.
    Includes bibliographical references and index.
    ISBN 978-1-59120-272-1
    1. Middle-aged men—Health and hygiene. 2. Older people—Health and age management. 3. Inflammation—Diet therapy. 4. Glycemic index.
5. Self-care, Health. I. Title.
    RA777.5.S556   2009
    613'.04234—dc22

                                                          2009044546

Editor: John Anderson
Typesetting/Book design: Gary A. Rosenberg
Cover design: Mike Stromberg

Printed in the United States of America

10 9 8 7 6 5 4 3 2 1

Contents

To my three sons—Ryan, Justin, and Dylan—
may each of you remain a WellMan!

And to Pam,
for your enduring support.

Acknowledgments

I would like to thank those who have contributed to *WellMan*. First, the team at Eternity Medicine Institute, who I hope will continue to help transform the health of men (and women) in the years ahead. Second, Randi Katz, Nadine Knowles, Peter Walker (photography), Gary Rosenberg (graphic design), and John Anderson, my editor, for keeping me on track.

A special thanks to my colleague from Cenegenics, Dr. Jacob Rosenstein, who was a patient of mine. In addition to his neurosurgery practice, he is now a Cenegenics affiliate and is helping other men transform their health. My thanks also to Cicely Valenti for the excellent information on exercise and to Marcus Niemo, my trainer.

I am also grateful to Scott Christian and Peter Derkx, for their introduction of healthy LIV Water to the U.S., and to Drs. Robert and Jack Slovak for their introduction of Marine Plasma. Simple innovative solutions like these, together with Peter Taunton's great Snap Fitness franchise, create an ideal environment for men to stay strong and healthy. Snap Fitness is now in most cities across America.

Finally, thanks to my publisher, Norman Goldfind, for recognizing the importance of "andropause" affecting more than 40 million men in the U.S. We now know that middle-aged men can reinvent themselves with the program outlined in *WellMan* so they can enjoy optimum health and vitality well into their nineties and beyond.

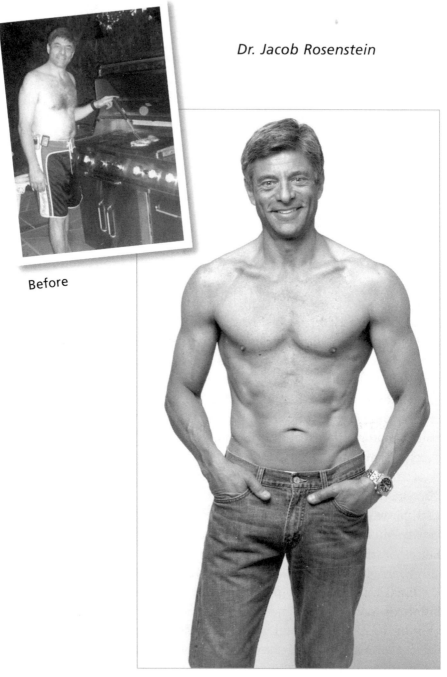

Dr. Jacob Rosenstein

Before

After

Foreword

As a long-time fitness industry veteran, I've seen people's opinions change considerably when it comes to health and wellness. When I first got started in the fitness business twenty years ago, my motivation was simple: to provide men and women of all ages with a high-quality exercise option that would allow them to look and feel better. The challenge, however, was that many believed that living a healthy lifestyle was more of a luxury than a necessity.

In 2003, I decided that a change was in order. I stripped down the big-box health club model that had dominated the industry for decades and created a more compact, state-of-the-art fitness facility that offered convenience and affordability without compromising the quality of the member experience. Snap Fitness has become the fastest-growing fitness franchise in the world, an accomplishment I attribute to people's ever-changing attitudes about the positive benefits of regular exercise and a generally more health-conscious society.

Today, I see the same change in public perception in the field of wellness and age management. A few years ago, if someone was speaking to me about "age management" or "anti-aging," the first thing I would have thought of is the cosmetic benefits. However, as I've become more familiar with this concept—and, more specifically, with the Integral Health Program presented in this book—I realize that the positive impact of age management programs reach much further than appearance.

As we look toward the future and examine the state of healthcare in this country, there are many variables affecting rising healthcare costs. Wellness and age management programs are helping to control these costs and will continue to do so in the coming years, thanks to the added longevity they provide consumers. I can speak to the benefits of the Integral Health Program, as it has helped me establish an even healthier lifestyle, allowing me to feel better than ever before.

Twenty years ago, many consumers looked at fitness as a benefit targeted at a select demographic, and age management and wellness programs are encountering this same challenge today. Just as physical fitness has proven to be a staple of living a long and healthy life, so too will these types of programs. You can learn more about the integral methodology in *WellMan* and see for yourself what makes it one of the most comprehensive age management programs available. Experience the benefits today of what will surely become a health and wellness staple of tomorrow.

—Peter Taunton,
Founder and CEO,
Snap Fitness

INTRODUCTION

At the Crossroads

I, LIKE MANY OF YOU, AM A MIDDLE-AGED MAN. I have had the opportunity of working as a primary care physician for many years. In this position, I came to recognize that health and disease are largely a matter of lifestyle, a choice we make every day on the road of life. For the past several years, my staff and I have worked exclusively in age management medicine and helped many patients take control of their health and delay, or even reverse, the course of degenerative disease. A focus on prevention and an integrated health program allows men to enjoy a longer life with greater vitality, passion, and meaning.

You have a choice to make. Many of you have reached a crossroads in your life. You can continue your current lifestyle with those extra pounds, decreased energy, lessened mental clarity, and that decreasing libido, or you can choose to reinvent yourself, becoming a "WellMan" full of renewed energy and passion, with a greater sense of well-being. We are not prisoners of our genetic destiny.

Medicine is now beginning to recognize that the key to successful aging is the control of "silent inflammation." Most of us have some idea of what inflammation is: if a wound gets hot, turns red, hurts, and swells, we recognize inflammation is at work. In this instance, inflammation is a beneficial process, serving to localize the area of injury as the immune system mobilizes to heal. But there's another kind of inflammation, silent inflammation, which has a more insidious nature—it goes on inside us year after year and can only be assessed by special blood tests. Researchers now recognize that silent inflammation is responsible for most chronic disease, including heart disease, Alzheimer's disease, and cancer. In fact, silent inflammation is now understood as the primary cause of aging itself.

THE INTEGRAL HEALTH PROGRAM

The Integral Health Program is the most advanced and comprehensive program currently available. In order to assess your pattern of health or disease, you need to look "under the water" at your lifestyle, culture, and worldview (see page 3). Unlike most medicine that looks only at the UR quadrant (see page 4), the Integral Health Model looks at all four quadrants. In this book, I will be sharing the knowledge we have gained over the past two decades to help you look and feel great.

In our Eternity Medicine Institutes, this consists of a three-step process designed to square the usual aging process for each individual (see page 5).

- Step One: MEASURE—Measuring includes a four-quadrant meta-analysis, a head-to-toe physical examination and over 250 individual biomarkers that together will assess your current health status.

- Step Two: MENTOR—The powerful Integral Health Program outlined in this book provides a comprehensive way of controlling silent inflammation and allows each individual to optimize their health. An added bonus to extending your health span is that you will be able to take full advantage of future medical breakthroughs that could result in increasing your longevity even further.

- Step Three: MONITOR—We also use advanced methods for recording, follow-up, and ongoing evaluation, the Lifetime Health Assessment and Monitoring Program (LHAMP). Our patients have access to their own test results, coaching from knowledgeable health professionals, and access to the latest wellness and age management science and products. Thirty of the world's most respected health professionals serve as the medical advisors to Eternity Medicine Institutes.

We believe that programs such as this will become part of the wellness revolution in the years ahead. How else will we be able to prevent the more than 1 million new cases of diabetes that will be diagnosed this year? Diabetes costs the United States close to $800

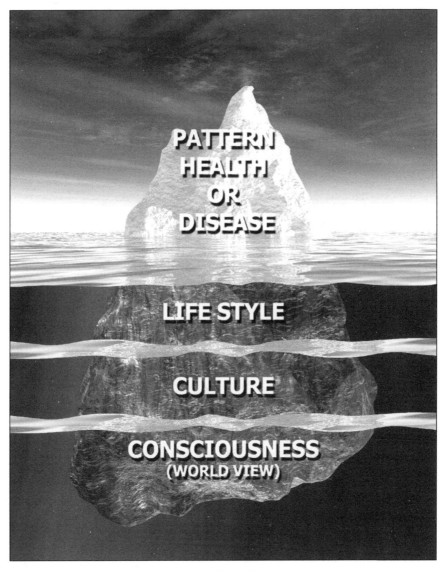

Integral Health

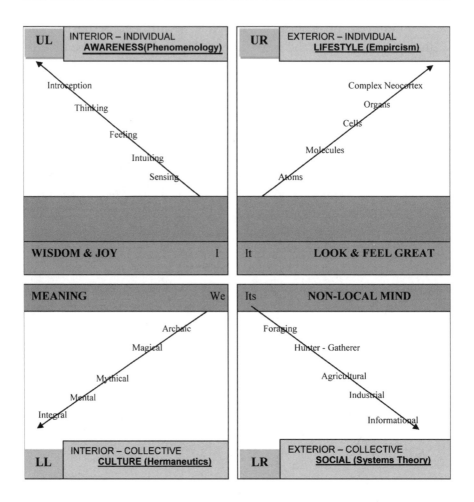

UL The interior of the individual. Our own immediate thoughts, feelings, sensations, and awareness (psycho-spiritual).

UR What any event looks like from the outside. Includes physical behavior, matter, energy, and the concrete body (biological).

LL The inside awareness of the group, its worldview, shared values (culture), and meaning (interpersonal).

LR The exterior forms and behavior of the group (social systems). This includes the environment (worldly).

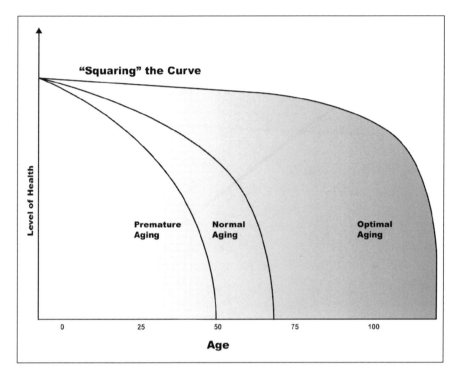

WellMan Health Span

billion per year. Diabetes alone could bankrupt our healthcare system. Similar grim statistics apply to obesity, heart disease and cancer.

The focus of this book is on men's health rather than the larger issues currently affecting the health-care industry, but they are clearly intimately connected. A focus on men's health and longevity is long overdue. Join this exciting journey to help you regain your health and vitality. I have not only done this for my clients but also for myself: I entered middle-age overweight and out of shape, with increasing sugar intolerance (pre-diabetes), hypertension, lacking both energy and drive, and experiencing falling libido. Within just three months, I was back on top of my game. I want to share my experience and knowledge with each of you.

Welcome to *WellMan*!

CHAPTER 1

Inflammation Control

Instead of different treatments for heart disease,
Alzheimer's, and colon cancer, there might be a single
inflammation remedy that would prevent all three.
—*TIME* MAGAZINE COVER STORY (FEBRUARY 23, 2004)

INFLAMMATION IS NOW UNDERSTOOD TO BE at the center of a wide range of conditions, from heart disease and hypertension to obesity and diabetes; from Alzheimer's and Parkinson's disease to depression, cancer, and arthritis. In fact, research shows that all chronic disease has a significant inflammatory component. Even aging itself appears to result from the cumulative effects of silent inflammation (what I call Inflam-Aging). When you consider how many of our aging population are affected with one or more chronic diseases (70 percent of Americans are overweight), you can begin to get an idea of the epidemic of inflammation we face today. I believe that this epidemic of silent inflammation is the single biggest factor responsible for our current health-care crisis. Our $2 trillion health-care bill (as large as the entire economy of China) is nearly 20 percent of our whole economy. But this silent inflammation remains largely unrecognized by physicians, patients, and other key stakeholders in the health-care system.

Although silent inflammation can cause a variety of disorders, many of us (and this, unfortunately, includes many physicians) do not know the warning signs of this kind of inflammation or the best way to treat it. This knowledge is critical because if a person has one inflammatory condition, the odds that he or she will develop another condition increase dramatically. Researchers have discovered, for example, that a man with rheumatoid arthritis has a 100 percent increased risk of a heart attack.[1] And other recent research has demonstrated that a high C-reactive protein (CRP) level, in addition to being a risk factor for heart disease, is also associated with age-related macular degeneration. Slowing down this chronic inflammation is vital to successful aging, so it is crucial for us to understand its manifestations and causes and then take the necessary measures to stop it.

Silent inflammation attacks the single layer of cells—the endothelium—that line the 50,000 miles of blood vessels within each of us, hence its widespread effects. For example, inflammation in the brain can cause depression, Alzheimer's disease, or attention deficit disorder (ADD); if the vessels to the heart are involved, a heart attack could result; erectile dysfunction may be the manifestation if the blood vessels to the penis have silent inflammation.

I will first look at the various manifestations of silent inflammation, from heart disease to aging itself. Next, I will discuss the primary causes of inflammation and ask "Are you inflamed?" You will then be ready to take control of silent inflammation.

MANIFESTATIONS OF SILENT INFLAMMATION

Heart and Blood Vessels

More than 2,000 people die each day in the United States from cardiovascular disease. Not long ago, most physicians thought of heart attacks as primarily a plumbing problem: over the years, fatty deposits would slowly build up on the insides of the major coronary arteries until they cut off the supply of blood to the heart. Low-density lipoprotein (LDL), the so-called "bad cholesterol," was thought to provide the raw material for these deposits. (I will show in Chapter 2 just how wrong this cholesterol-heart hypothesis is.) The problem is that more than half of all heart attacks occur in people with normal cholesterol levels.[2] Not only that, doctors also find that the most dangerous deposits (plaque) aren't necessarily all that large.

In the 1990s, Paul Ridker, M.D., of Brigham and Women's Hospital, in Boston, became convinced that some type of inflammatory reaction was responsible for the rupturing plaques. Dr. Ridker used CRP (discovered more than twenty years ago), a molecule produced by the liver in response to inflammation, as the marker. By 1997, he had shown that healthy middle-aged men with the highest CRP levels were three times more likely to suffer a heart attack in the next six years compared to those with the lowest CRP levels.[3]

Of all the many factors that are found in both our internal and external environments, it is primarily our diet with its excessive amounts of high-glycemic carbohydrates that sets the stage for silent inflammation (see Chapter 2). Let us explore some of the other factors responsible for producing "fire in the heart."

Heavy Metals

There are numerous published reports describing adverse clinical effects with aluminum, cadmium, copper, iron, lead, and mercury. According to data from the U.S. Toxics Release Inventory, in the year 2000 industry in the United States released 4.3 million pounds of mercury compounds into the environment and generated 4.9 million pounds of mercury compounds in toxic waste.[4] This toxic metal burden increases low-grade inflammation at the cellular level, which interferes with mitochondrial function (cellular energy production), and therefore has a negative effect on the endocrine (glandular), immune, and metabolic systems.

The cardiovascular system is extraordinarily sensitive to mercury. In one small study of thirteen patients with idiopathic dilated cardiomyopathy (a deterioration of heart muscle function), investigators found mean mercury concentrations in excess of 22,000 times normal.[5] Higher mercury levels were thus implicated as causes of this form of cardiomyopathy.

How do we become mercury toxic in the first place? Quite simply: breathing bad air and eating bad fish. Most mercury vapors arise in the atmosphere from the industrialization of coal. Mercury is then inhaled into the lungs and transmitted to tissues. The precipitation of mercury vapors in the water supply is another important factor.

Rainfall precipitates mercury into ponds, lakes, and streams. Bacteria and algae sequester mercury, small (bait) fish ingest algae-laden methylmercury, and then the bigger fish eat these smaller fish. And the larger the fish, the more time it has had to accumulate mercury from its diet of smaller fish. When we enjoy a dinner with a mercury-overloaded fish (sea bass and grouper have the most mercury), that heavy metal has made it into our food chain.

Researchers studied the association between fish intake and myocardial infarction (heart attack) using hair analysis and urinary excretion to measure mercury levels in 1,833 men. Their results showed that men with the highest levels of hair mercury content had twice the incidence of acute myocardial infarction and almost three times the incidence of cardiovascular death as those with lower hair mercury content.[6] Both hair and urinary mercury increase oxidized LDL, and high levels of oxidized LDL prime the pump for further inflammation.

Although somewhat controversial, dental amalgams ("mercury" fillings) are another source of unwanted mercury toxins in the body. The removal of old amalgams by a biological dentist should be strongly considered by anyone with signs and symptoms of mercury overload, such as headache, tremor, cardiac disease of unknown etiology, confusion, weakness, weight loss, insomnia, joint pain, and fatigue, to mention a few.

The easiest way to diagnose heavy metal toxicity is to ingest a dose of oral DMSA (dimercaptosuccinic acid) and collect the urine for six hours. In my practice, I commonly perform this test on patients with unexplained fatigue, fibromyalgia, and neurological and emotional problems, in addition to cardiac disease.

Free Radicals

Free radicals are highly reactive, imbalanced molecules produced during oxidation that steal electrons from cells to neutralize their charge. Free radicals interfere with enzymatic reactions and cause significant metabolic stress, damaging cells and DNA. Oxidation may occur within the body through simple metabolic processes like eating, drinking, and breathing, which generate free radicals as byproducts of cellular energy production. Alcohol, drugs, poor diets, radiation, and other catalysts all accelerate the production of free radicals in the body. The danger of free radicals is that they fan the fires of inflammation and attack cell membranes, ultimately disrupting cellular communication. When free radical damage disturbs the integrity of cell membranes, they leak and excessive waste builds up inside the cells.

One of the primary ways we can protect ourselves from free radical damage is to take antioxidants. Because cell membranes are composed mostly of fat, fat-soluble antioxidants like alpha-lipoic acid, coenzyme Q_{10}, and vitamin E can best penetrate into the cell. Antioxidants slow the aging process by promoting cellular repair, inhibiting inflammation, and preventing production of the inflammatory substances that accelerate aging. Many antioxidants also actively block the oxidation of LDL that contributes to silent inflammation and need to be part of your advanced supplementation program.

Nanobacteria

Although oxidized LDL cholesterol helps to set the stage for atherosclerosis, there are other inflammatory causes of cardiovascular disease. Nanobacteria may well be an important initiating event behind atherosclerosis. Nanobacteria are so minute that they eluded researchers for decades. They're a hundredth the size of normal bacteria, and until recently, nobody believed that anything so small could even be alive. It turns out, however, that nanobacteria are not only very vital and thriving, but may cause damage to our health.

Scientists from the Hungarian Academy of Sciences have reported finding nanobacteria in more than 60 percent of carotid artery-clogging plaques studied.[7] They also validated previous research reports of how truly minuscule these bacteria are, and how easily they can enter the body via blood exchange and blood products. Nanobacteria have a protective calcified coat that makes them highly resistant to heat, radiation, and all antibiotics except tetracycline. Nanobacteria have also been implicated in nephrolithiasis (kidney stones) and polycystic kidney disease.

More research will be needed to determine whether or not nanobacteria are a real culprit behind coronary arteriosclerosis. For now, it is prudent to keep in mind that microbes could play a substantial factor in the genesis of silent inflammation.

Spirochetes

In 1982, Willy Burgdorfer, Ph.D., discovered the cause of Lyme disease when he isolated spirochetes of the genus *Borrelia* from the midgut of *Ixodes* ticks. Some researchers believe that as many as 60 million people in the U.S. are infected with *Borrelia*, but that Lyme disease occurs only when their immune systems become overloaded. Lyme disease has been reported in forty-seven states and on four continents, and ticks are not the only source. Blood transfusions, fleas, mosquitoes, sexual intercourse, and unpasteurized cow's and goat's milk have also transmitted the disease. People with Lyme disease are often simultaneously co-infected with other viruses and bacteria.

The spirochetes responsible for Lyme disease do best in an anaerobic (low-oxygen) environment and cannot tolerate large quantities of oxygen. They can change their shape and chemical structure and are more evolved than bacteria in many ways. Furthermore, these spirochetes can turn off several surface proteins, which has the effect of keeping the immune system from detecting them. This stealth-type camouflage prevents antibodies from attaching to them, and prevents the enzymes in the blood from finding and destroying them. In this way, the spirochete can penetrate virtually any tissue in our body, including blood vessels, heart, brain, and oral cavity.

Periodontal Disease

Multiple microbes, including spirochetes, bacteria, and viruses, can be cultured in and around the teeth and periodontal sections in the oral cavity. There is a significant relationship between gum disease and chronic inflammation. Low-grade inflammation, particularly in periodontal areas, can cause immune system decline and raise CRP levels. In one study of fifty patients referred for angiography and assessed for periodontal disease, there was a significant relationship between the extent of coronary atherosclerosis and periodontal disease. Periodontal disease may increase the risk of cardiovascular disease by 20 percent.[8] Cardiologists are especially cognizant of the relationship between oral hygiene, edentulous teeth, gum disease, halitosis, and a strong probability of subsequent cardiovascular disease. Practicing good oral hygiene and taking antioxidants, colloidal silver, magnesium, essential fatty acids, and coenzyme Q_{10} can help support gum health, thereby reducing chronic inflammation.

Toxic Blood Syndrome

Many heart attacks and strokes occur when arteries are narrowed by only a third, so it's not the blood vessels that are of interest to us but the blood *flow* when it's compromised by plaque rupture. Inflammation is the primary culprit responsible for vascular disease. In fact, 95 percent of chronically sick patients have abnormally high blood coagulation.[9] Many of these patients have "toxic blood syndrome," characterized by elevated levels of oxidized LDL, C-reactive protein, fibrinogen, homocysteine, lipoprotein(a), and ferritin. Elevated CRP was the most significant of twelve markers in 28,263 healthy postmenopausal women as a predictor of future cardiac events. It was the strongest risk factor associated with an acute coronary event such as plaque rupture and heart attack.

Homocysteine

High levels of the amino acid homocysteine is a risk factor for cardiovascular disease, and it's also been implicated in osteoporosis, macular degeneration, migraines, low birth weight, neural tube defects, some cancers, and Alzheimer's disease. Homocysteine is directly toxic to blood vessels in the brain and heart. Elevated levels wreak oxidative stress and cause endothelial dysfunction, neuronal DNA damage, and mitochondrial membrane weakening. High homocysteine levels in the brain cause cerebral microangiopathy and apoptosis (programmed cell death) of neural cells.

Hyperhomocysteinemia has been shown to double the incidence of Alzheimer's disease. In one study of 1,092 people who were "dementia free" over an eight-year follow-up, 111 developed dementia and 83 developed full-blown Alzheimer's disease. Those with homocysteine levels above 14 mmol/L doubled their risk, and for every 5 mmol/L increase, their risk for Alzheimer's disease rose by 40 percent.[10]

One of the most important factors in lowering homocysteine is the use of various B vitamin components, including folic acid, calcium folinate, vitamins B_6 and B_{12}, pyridoxal phosphate, and betaine hydrochloride (trimethylglycine). Garlic, beets, broccoli, and S-adenosyl-methionine (SAMe) are also potent methyl donors, helpful in reversing toxic homocysteine back to harmless methionine. Recently, researchers found that a new bioactive form of folate—5-methyl-tetrahydro folate (5-MTHF)—which, given to patients with coronary disease, resulted in a 700 percent higher plasma folate level compared with folic acid.

A homocysteine level less than 7 mmol/L is ideal. Levels over 10 mmol/L are unacceptable, especially in those with presenile dementia or arteriosclerotic cardiovascular disease. High homocysteine levels are treacherous, especially in the company of elevated lipoprotein(a) because together they can induce the binding of Lp(a) to fibrin, a clot-promoting mechanism. I have seen elevated homocysteine in the company of high Lp(a) in many of my patients who have heart disease, and treat it aggressively.

Lipoprotein(a)

Lp(a) is a cholesterol particle that is highly inflammatory and thrombotic (induces clot formation). In a ten-year study of myocardial infarction in 5,200 participants, those with the highest Lp(a) levels had a 70 percent increased incidence of myocardial infarction.[11] For the clinical cardiologist, Lp(a) is a difficult risk factor to neutralize, because statin therapy for treating high cholesterol is known to increase Lp(a). Recently, the herb *Ginkgo biloba* has been used with good results in decreasing Lp(a). I have found that other targeted nutraceuticals, especially liver-supporting nutrients, coenzyme Q_{10}, policosanol (a natural extract of plant waxes), and omega-3 essential fatty acids (fish oils), in combination with niacin (vitamin B_3) will often neutralize the toxic effects of Lp(a). Advanced lipid testing is an essential component of age management medicine.

Fibrinogen

Fibrinogen is a coagulation protein. Levels greater than 360 mg/dl are undesirable and have been associated with coronary calcification. Abnormally elevated levels have been observed in smokers and postmenopausal women with increasing frequency. Fish oils, garlic, bromelain (from pineapple), and natural COX-2 inhibitors (anti-inflammatory substances) such as ginger and green tea will help to alleviate high fibrinogen.

Ferritin

High levels of serum ferritin (stored iron) are associated with increased risk for myocardial infarction. The high levels of iron that can oxidize LDL cholesterol may reflect iron overload or hereditary hemochromatosis (a disorder of iron metabolism). In the setting of high iron overload, it is important to cut iron consumption to a minimum and use high-dose vitamin C with caution, as megadoses of greater than 500 mg daily may enhance iron absorption from the diet.

In summary, it's important to assess all these "toxic blood" components, particularly in an individual with a family history of early-onset, or premature, cardiovascular disease. The assessment of arteriosclerosis needs to go beyond cholesterol and triglyceride monitoring, and these inflammatory and thrombotic components are the most undesirable factors in the generation and promotion of plaque.

Younger plaque is soft and covered by a thin fibrous cap, loaded with cholesterol, and it's quite volatile. This young plaque often goes unnoticed on angiograms. To some extent, many of us have atherosclerosis—the real question is, "Do you have an unstable plaque?" Inside fatty plaques, macrophages can become engorged and incompetent to do their job. Instead, they evolve into foam cells, releasing pro-inflammatory toxic substances that may result in further instability to the plaque.

It used to be thought that cholesterol was the major marker for atherosclerosis, but this is no longer the case. In fact, triglycerides (the other blood fat made by your liver from a high-carbohydrate diet) is far more predictive of heart disease than cholesterol. Pro-inflammatory messengers, cytokines and leukotrienes, are now recognized as behind-the-scenes culprits together with sugar and insulin. When inflammation is present, cytokines instruct the liver to increase intermediary inflammatory substances, such as CRP, that are released into the blood and serve as measures of underlying chronic inflammation. By interrupting and arresting inflammation, we can help to prevent atherosclerosis, hypertension, heart disease, stroke, and even sudden death.

Obesity, Metabolic Syndrome, and Diabetes Mellitus

Obesity

By definition, a person is obese when he or she is thirty or more pounds over his or her ideal weight. Nearly 70 percent of Americans are overweight and there are now more obese than overweight Americans. In fact, close to 2 million Americans weigh more than 500 pounds—the super obese. Nearly 20 percent of children are now overweight; for the first time in human history, children may have a shorter life expectancy than their parents because of obesity-related illnesses. The health consequences of this have nearly overtaken tobacco as the number one risk factor in America. Being overweight is the primarly disease risk factor for developing type 2 diabetes. The prevalence of type 2 diabetes mellitus in children has increased twenty-five times since 1950. In fact, a child born today will have a one in three chance of developing diabetes.[12] Thirty percent of obese children also have metabolic syndrome.

This excess weight results largely from the increased consumption of junk foods consisting chiefly of refined sugars, high-glycemic carbohydrates, and trans-fats (hydrogenated oils found in processed foods). High amounts of sugar and carbohydrates trigger increased insulin levels, which promote storage of fat. In fact, the greatest single change in the American diet is the spectacular increase in sugar consumption from less than 15 pounds per person per year in the 1820s, to 100 pounds by the 1920s, to over 150 pounds today![13]

Fat doesn't just hang and look unsightly—it is very metabolically active. In fact, fat produces an increase in a wide array of toxins (CRP, interleukin-6, adhesion molecules, cytokines, etc.) that produces even more inflammation.

Insulin resistance occurs when your cells become less responsive to the actions of insulin, forcing your pancreas to make even more insulin in an effort to drive sugar into your cells. This increase in insulin further increases storage of fat and increases obesity. The number one cause of liver disease in America, in fact, is obesity; this disease is called "fatty liver." So the real question behind our obesity epidemic is "What actually causes insulin resistance?" Researchers believe that the cause lies in the endothelial cells, the single layer of cells that line your blood vessels and separate the blood from your tissues. Endothelial dysfunction will prevent insulin (and other nutrients) from passing from the bloodstream to the receptors on the cell's surface, thus preventing the cell from taking up glucose. The body responds by pumping out even more insulin (hyperinsulinemia). The cause of this endothelial dysfunction may be silent inflammation. A study done at Louisiana State University showed that giving patients 1–8 grams of docosahexaenoic acid (DHA; a major

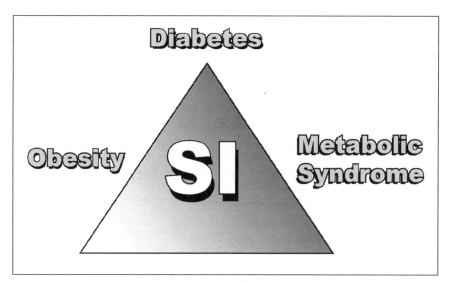

Silent Inflammation at the Center of Common Chronic Diseases

component of fish oil) for twelve weeks decreased insulin resistance by 70 percent.[14]

To prove that silent inflammation precedes insulin resistance, researchers ran a pilot study on pediatric obesity patients. The children were divided into two groups, both of which had high scores on a silent inflammation profile (SIP), a screening test that measures markers for inflammation. Both groups got the same diet, but only one group received a tablespoon of fish oil containing eicosapentaenoic acid (EPA) and DHA. If silent inflammation was causing insulin resistance, then the group that got the fish oil should do better than the other group. This is exactly what happened; as their profile scores dropped, so did their weight.[15] This suggests that silent inflammation may be the underlying cause of insulin resistance and therefore obesity. This means that unless you treat this silent inflammation, it will be very difficult to lose weight.

Metabolic Syndrome
(Syndrome X or Insulin Resistance Syndrome)

More than 40 percent of adults over the age of forty now suffer from metabolic syndrome.[16] The World Health Organization (WHO) diagnostic criteria for metabolic syndrome include:

- Hyperinsulinemia or fasting glucose >110 mg/dl and two out of the following:

  1. Abdominal obesity—waist/hip ratio of 7.9, or body mass index (BMI) greater than 30, or waist circumference over 40 inches in men or over 35 inches in women.

  2. Serum triglycerides greater than 150 mg/dl and high-density lipoprotein (HDL) cholesterol less than 35 mg/dl.

  3. Blood pressure higher than 140/90.

The main problem is that when skeletal muscle resists insulin-mediated uptake of glucose, clinically defined insulin resistance occurs. When insulin resistance occurs, long-term glucose levels do not necessarily rise because the pancreas generates more insulin. The maintenance of normal glucose via increased insulin production (hyperinsulinemia) is the fundamental metabolic disturbance underlying metabolic syndrome. The fall in insulin secretion leading to hyperglycemia (diabetes) occurs as a late phenomenon, often 7–10 years later.

Metabolic syndrome is a recipe for increased risk of cardiovascular disease (six-fold higher) and diabetes with all its associated increased mortality and morbidity. Metabolic syndrome has overtaken cigarette smoking as the number one risk factor for heart disease among the U.S. population.

Diabetes

Diabetes has become a national epidemic. More money is spent on the complications of diabetes than on any other chronic disease—the U.S. spent close to $800 billion on diabetes care in 2008.[17] Over 1 million new cases of diabetes were diagnosed in 2008 alone. There is a five- to ten-fold decrease in life expectancy with diabetes, and an increased risk of stroke and heart disease (75 percent of diabetics will die of coronary artery disease).

There are two major types of diabetes. Type 1 diabetes (juvenile) usually occurs in younger persons and results from a complete shutdown of the pancreas with no insulin production. This results from some environmental trigger that sets up an autoimmune reaction that wipes out the pancreas so that the person is required to inject insulin each day. More than 90 percent of all diabetics have type 2 diabetes. As mentioned earlier, silent inflammation appears to cause endothelial dysfunction that produces insulin resistance. Insulin resistance in turn causes the pancreas to secrete more insulin (hyperinsulinemia) in an effort to reduce blood sugar levels. Eventually the pancreas burns out and glucose begins to rise to dangerous levels. This increased glucose produces free radicals (oxidative stress) and is neurotoxic to the brain. Hyperinsulinemia usually precedes the development of type 2 diabetes by about eight years, but they both result from increased insulin resistance.

Silent inflammation is at the center of obesity, metabolic syndrome, and diabetes. The most critical factor in reducing inflammation is loss of excess weight. A weight loss of as little as 5 percent can significantly reduce fasting glucose, insulin, and inflammatory markers. Fish oil and other phytonutrients, coupled with a Paleolithic diet (the original human diet), will reverse silent inflammation, obesity, metabolic syndrome, and diabetes.

Cancer

Cancer refers to the growth of abnormal cells. Although some cancers affect children, they are usually age related: the older you are, the greater your risk of cancer. Cancers are caused by mutations in our cells' genetic blueprint or DNA (deoxyribonucleic acid). These mutations occur in two ways: through random transcriptional error when cells replicate or through free radical damage to DNA. The immune system usually destroys abnormal cells, but as we age our surveillance is not as competent. Cancer is the second leading cause of death: more than 500,000 people die each year from the various forms of cancer due to this "immune-o-pause."

According to researchers, more than 50 percent of all cancers are related to chronic inflammation or chronic infections.[18] Both cause free radicals, which can damage DNA. Epidemiological studies have also linked hyperinsulinemia, which causes inflammation, to an increased risk of breast, prostate, colorectal, and endometrial cancers.

High-dose fish oil has been found to decrease metastasis (spread of tumors), increase apoptosis (cell death in tumors), and reduce angiogenesis (blood cell formation by tumors). Fish oil will also decrease sugar and insulin levels, helping to slow tumor growth (blood sugar feeds tumor cells and excess insulin encourages them to divide). It is well known that women who eat the highest amount of fish are least likely to develop breast cancer. Cancer prevention is all about reducing silent inflammation.

In his book *Good Calories, Bad Calories*, Gary Taubes cites several interesting epidemiological studies. First, in the 1950s, epidemiologist John Higginson studied cancer in native African populations and compared them with the incidence in the U.S. With a few exceptions, cancer in African natives was remarkably uncommon. This led him to conclude that most human cancers were caused by environmental factors and that diet and lifestyle factors were the primary suspects. It appears that once more than 80 pounds of sugar is consumed by a person each year, the incidence of cancer increases dramatically.

In 1981, Oxford epidemiologists Richard Doll and Richard Peto concluded that at least 75–80 percent of cancers in the U.S. might be avoidable with appropriate changes in diet and lifestyle.[19] Researchers had previously noted that the five nations with the highest breast cancer mortality in women in the late 1970s included the United Kingdom, the Netherlands, Ireland, Denmark, and Canada, which had the highest sugar consumption in the same descending order; those countries with the lowest mortality rates—Japan, Yugoslavia, Portugal, Spain, and Italy—had the lowest sugar consumption. Other researchers have shown that tumors will burn perhaps thirty times as much blood sugar as normal cells, and insulin acts as a promoter of growth and proliferation in healthy and malignant cells.

Finally, a more recent landmark study linked being overweight with higher cancer risk. "Food, Nutrition, and the Prevention of Cancer: A Global Perspective," produced by the World Cancer Research Fund (WCRF) and the American Institute for Cancer Research (AICR), found that the impact of nutrition, physical activity, and body composition on the risk of cancer is much larger than even the researchers expected. As they stated, "People forget body fat is not an inert glob that we are carrying around on the waistline and thighs. It's a metabolically active tissue that produces substances (inflammation) in the body that promote the development of cancer."

Unfortunately, the typical American is consuming too many refined carbohydrates, saturated fats, and trans-fats, together with a huge intake of fructose—found in sodas and most packaged fast foods. The concern isn't as much about reducing red meat as it is about eating higher quality meats. For example, a person in Ethiopia may eat red meat, but it's goat, a lean red meat source. Here in the U.S., most people are choosing meats like sausage, bacon, cutlets, and processed lunchmeat, which should be replaced with chicken, fish, bison, and lean cuts of organic beef and pork. The key to preventing cancer is to eat the original human diet, the Paleolithic diet.

Immune System Dysfunction

Our body's immune system is a complex and elegant one designed to recognize and destroy any invader that has the potential to harm us. If an invader manages to penetrate our skin or mucous membranes and enter the bloodstream, the invader sets off a sophisticated alarm system. The surveillance white blood cells (WBCs) release their own on-site defenses but also send out chemical messages throughout the body asking for help and reinforcements.

WBCs are made up of a variety of cells that perform different functions. B lymphocytes act as the advance guard by making antibodies. Neutrophils have a short life and are very destructive. Macrophages ingest invaders and secrete enzymes that act as a clean-up team. T lymphocytes track down and destroy invaders that have escaped the bloodstream and are hiding in the tissues. Prostaglandins and leukotrienes are chemical messengers, made from a fatty acid called arachidonic acid, that play a crucial role in the inflammatory reaction. Normally, the invader is vanquished, healing of the tissues occurs, and life goes on.

Inflammatory disease is just an exaggeration of this normal immune system response. If the invader becomes chronic, there is a category of inflammatory disease called allergic disease. The body's own cells may also trigger this kind of over-response, and these conditions are called autoimmune diseases. Here, I list a number of these conditions.

Food Allergies: Various foods can maintain the body's inflammatory response at a high idle and exacerbate symptoms of other inflammatory diseases (asthma, rheumatoid arthritis) or raise blood pressure and blood sugar levels.

Nightshade Sensitivity: Some people, including an estimated 20 percent of people with rheumatoid arthritis, react to one or more nightshade foods (tomatoes, potatoes, eggplant, peppers, tomatillos, and tobacco).

Inhalant Allergies: Immune system overreactions can result from any type of innocuous substance, such as pollens, molds, and cat dander. It is estimated that 60 million Americans have allergies, allergic rhinitis being the most common. I believe that the key to effective treatment is a change in diet and select anti-inflammatory nutraceuticals.

Lupus Erythematosus: Lupus is an autoimmune disease that can affect the skin, joints, kidneys, lungs, and the cardiovascular system. Ninety percent of patients experience joint problems, rashes, and sensitivity to light. Connective tissue is the main target.

Multiple Sclerosis: MS is an autoimmune disease in which immune cells attack the myelin sheath around nerves. When the myelin becomes inflamed, patients develop weakness, difficulty walking, double vision, speech problems, and depression. MS affects over 500,000 Americans, generally between the ages of twenty and forty, and more women than men.

Asthma: During asthmatic episodes (attacks), the body's airways overact to pollen, dander, cigarette smoke, cold air, or other stimuli. The airway wall muscles begin to spasm, allowing less air to reach the lungs. An inflammatory response results in a rapid thickening of mucus, which further narrows the airway. Several decades ago, asthma was a rare disorder; today, it affects over 17 million Americans, one-third of them children.

Although many causes have been suggested, diet is not often mentioned. The modern diet, which is high in pro-inflammatory omega-6 fatty acids and trans-fats and low in antioxidants, sets the stage for asthmatic reactions. Several studies have shown that when both children and adults consume more fruits and vegetables (antioxidants), they are far less likely to wheeze. Other research points to the inadequate levels of omega-3 fatty acids in the diet. The increase in childhood asthma corresponds with a five-fold increase in the use of vegetable oils (rich in pro-inflammatory omega-6s and a shift to margarine instead of butter).[20] Vitamins C and E, beta carotene, and lycopene can ease reactions. In addition, omega-3s can reduce reactivity in asthmatics. Magnesium, boswellia, and pycnogenol also help. Researchers have mapped out at a cellular level how grains and dairy foods set the stage for many autoimmune diseases and how a return to our "original human diet" can help reverse these diseases.

Brain Disorders

Alzheimer's Disease (AD): AD is the most common type of dementia—estimates are that over 5 million Americans have some form of Alzheimer's. It is characterized by beta-amyloid protein accumulation in the brain, and free radicals stimulate formation of these amyloid plaques. The silent inflammation profile (SIP) scores of Alzheimer's patients are two times higher than normal. Common anti-inflammatory drugs have been shown to reduce the risk of AD.[21] Vitamins E and C, coenzyme Q_{10}, lipoic acid, acetyl-L-carnitine, turmeric, and fish oil have been shown effective in combating AD.

Attention Deficit Disorder (ADD): ADD afflicts about 3–5 percent of children. One factor common to all ADD patients is the deficiency of the neurotransmitter dopamine. The severity of ADD is directly related to the level of silent inflammation. It is important for them to eat a Paleolithic diet in addition to extra fish oil. Fish oil can help alleviate ADD because it decreases inflammation and increases dopamine levels;[22] children will often need up to 10–15 grams of fish oil per day to normalize their SIP scores.

Parkinson's Disease: Parkinson's has similarities to both Alzheimer's and ADD. It is an inflammatory condition in the substantia nigra (an area of gray matter in the midbrain) that is characterized by the loss of dopamine. High-dose fish oil and a Paleolithic diet are useful in treatment.

Depression: Depression has increased significantly over the last few decades. More than 20 million Americans suffer from depression. SIP scores correspond to the severity of depression. New Zealanders, who eat the least amount of fish in the industrialized world, have fifty times the rate of depression as the Japanese.[23] Fish oil also increases serotonin levels, a neurotransmitter that helps with depression.

Schizophrenia: These patients have very low levels of omega-3 fatty acids in their bloodstream. EPA has anti-inflammatory properties and DHA provides structural properties necessary for optimal brain function.[24] One needs to use both, and in high enough doses, for successful results.

Gastrointestinal Tract Diseases

Celiac Disease (Gluten Enteropathy): This disease appears to result from a genetic intolerance to a group of gliadins, gluten proteins found in wheat, barley, and rye. Exposure to these proteins results in chronic inflammation of the small intestinal villi, leading to malabsorption, diarrhea, and weight loss. A number of people who have "celiac genes" won't develop the disorder and not everyone with the disorder can be found to have the genes. It also does not explain the wide range of extra-gastrointestinal inflammatory conditions associated with gluten sensitivity, including dermatitis, thyroiditis, diabetes, and neurological dysfunction.

A closer look reveals that celiac disease results from a complex interaction between several genes, dietary gluten, and other environmental factors, one of which is the microbial ecology of the intestine. By seeing this as an inflammatory process rather than a "disease," the possibilities for real healing begins as we expand our thinking beyond simply eliminating gluten. You can restore the intestinal bacterial balance with probiotics (friendly bacteria) and enzymes, and you can begin to modify the inflammatory process with omega-3 and omega-5 fatty acids, antioxidants, and other anti-inflammatory phytochemicals.

Gastritis, Ulcers, and Stomach Cancer: *Helicobacter pylori* was recognized in the 1990s as the leading cause of gastritis, ulcers, and stomach cancer. *H. pylori* irritates the stomach wall, but the immune response to this infection causes most of the damage. White blood cells are mobilized to the site of infection, where they release free radicals and pro-inflammatory eicosanoids, such as prostaglandin E_2. *H. pylori* is highly resistant to this immune response, which can inflame the stomach wall and may lead to an ulcer. Free radicals damage the DNA in the stomach wall cells, increasing the chance of mutations, some of which could cause cancer. Vitamins B and C, carotenes, and antibiotics will usually cure the problem.

Inflammatory Bowel Disease (IBD): Ulcerative colitis and Crohn's disease are often difficult to distinguish. Ulcerative colitis is an inflammation limited to the wall of the colon. Abdominal cramps, fever, and bloody diarrhea are the primary symptoms. Similar symptoms, generally affecting the ileum without blood in the stools, is more suggestive of Crohn's disease. More than 1 million Americans have inflammatory bowel disease; it is more common in people of Jewish descent.

IBD appears to be increasing and seems to involve an abnormal activation of the immune system, an exaggerated immune response to normal constituents of the mucosal microflora. Changes in our diet and other environmental factors no longer provide the proper milieu for the gastrointestinal tract to properly activate the immune system. Prebiotics and probiotics can be very helpful for IBD. Omega-3 and omega-5 fatty acids, antioxidants, and a Paleolithic diet can also help control this disease.

Leaky Gut Syndrome: In a normal, healthy intestine, the tight cell junctions constitute a barrier that provides limited access for substances from the lumen to be absorbed inside the body. In an unhealthy (inflamed) intestine, these tight junctions become "leaky" and large molecules (including amino acids with antigenic sites) can slip into the circulation. Drugs, an unhealthy diet, infections, and alcohol can all influence the permeability of the gut. These absorbed substances can trigger further inflammation resulting in abnormal immune reactions throughout the body. The supplement SeaVive (Roper Nutrition) contains high-quality fish proteins that can be utilized by sick intestinal cells to help leaky gut syndrome.

Bone, Joint, and Connective Tissue Disorders

More than 50 percent of Americans over the age of sixty-five have some degree of osteoarthritis. In this disorder, there is a gradual degeneration of the cartilage that lines the joints, bringing pain, swelling, and restricted movement. The underlying problem is inflammation. Rheumatoid arthritis is an autoimmune disease that commonly begins between the ages of thirty and fifty. It is three times more common in women than men and may run in families. In this condition, the body produces antibodies that attack its own tissues (the synovial membrane in joints) and causes severe inflammation. More than 2 million Americans suffer from rheumatoid arthritis.

Fibromyalgia is a form of chronic rheumatism (a condition affecting the muscles, ligaments, and other connective tissue) characterized by widespread pain, fatigue, and sleep disturbance, and it is surprisingly common and debilitating. It is more common in women than men and can affect children, sometimes as young as eight years old. Restless leg syndrome (RLS) may occur in half of fibromyalgia patients. Again, inflammation appears to be the final common pathway resulting in most of the symptoms.

Sarcopenia is the result of a 40 percent total decrease in muscle size between 24–80 years of age. New research findings suggest inflammation may be an important cause of muscle loss, resulting in disability in old age. There are also higher rates of osteoporosis, insulin resistance, obesity, and arthritis among those with sarcopenia.

All of these conditions can be helped by avoiding certain foods (such as the nightshade family of vegetables) and reducing exposure to certain chemical substances (organic solvents) and infectious agents (Epstein-Barr virus, mycoplasma). In addition to detoxification and the Paleolithic diet, there are many nutraceuticals that can decrease the inflammation even more, such as glucosamine and chondroitin, methylsulfonylmethane (MSM; a sulfur compound), niacinamide (vitamin B_3), and the amino acid tryptophan. Herbs such as turmeric, ginger, and boswellia will also help control the inflammation. Omega-3 fish oil and omega-5s can be very helpful; both need to be taken in sufficient quantities (at least 5 grams per day) to have maximum results.

Aging-Associated Problems

We do not die of old age. We die from a host of degenerative diseases. Anything that raises insulin will increase silent inflammation, which will hasten cardiovascular disease, cancer, Alzheimer's—in short, physical degeneration and aging itself. "Anything that raises blood sugar—in particular, the consumption of refined and easily digestible carbohydrates—will increase the generation of oxidants and free radicals; it will increase the rate of oxidative stress and glycation, and the formation and accumulation of advanced glycation end-products (AGEs)," writes Gary Taubes.[25]

Taubes notes that there is a prevalent myth that the causes of obesity and the common chronic diseases (and aging) are complex and thus no simple answer is possible. In fact, diet and sedentary lifestyles are critical in causing most of the diseases of civilization, particularly excess weight. "Weight (inflammation) sits like a spider at the center of an intricate, tangled web of health and disease," wrote Harvard epidemiologist Walter Willett, in his book *Eat, Drink and Be Healthy*.[26] This excess weight and its principal cause—a diet rich in refined and easily digestible carbohydrates—is the simple answer. The result is chronic hyperinsulinemia and inflammation. When this primary cause of inflammation is coupled with the other environmental causes I have previously covered, you begin to see how chronic disease and aging in men is mostly due to excessive "silent inflammation" and not due to your genes.

THE PRIMARY CAUSE OF INFLAMMATION

Our Paleolithic ancestors' diet contained roughly equal parts of omega-3 and omega-6 fatty acids. Today, we consume more than twenty times as much omega-6 as we do omega-3. As a result, our bodies tend to produce an over-abundance of pro-inflammatory prostaglandins and a paucity of anti-inflammatory prostaglandins.

—MONICA REINAGEL, *THE INFLAMMATION-FREE DIET PLAN* (2006)

Physicians since ancient times have recognized the importance of inflammation in health and disease. The Latin terminology handed down from classical medicine describes the cardinal features of inflammation: *rubor* (redness), *tumor* (swelling), *calor* (heat), and *dolor* (pain). Roman physician Galen (129–200 A.D.) added a fifth sign, *functio laesa* (disturbed function). Two centuries later it was proposed that excessive secretion (*fluor*) should also be added. Most of these signs of inflammation relate to alterations in the vascular (blood vessel) system. As I have shown, inflammation and the endothelium are intimately connected.

Knowledge about the cellular basis of inflammation had to wait for advances in light microscopy made in the nineteenth century. The research of Rudolf Virchow (1821–1902), among others, led to the recognition of the role of leukocytes (white blood cells) and host defenses against foreign bodies or microbes. The molecular nature of the messages exchanged between cells during inflammatory reactions was developed largely during the twentieth century. Advances in molecular biology led to the important discovery of how histamine, prostaglandins, leukotrienes, and cytokines, among others, were involved in inflammation. More recently, we have recognized that many cell types, including vascular, endothelial, and smooth-muscle cells, can produce and respond to various inflammatory signals.

The immune system's ability to mount an adequate inflammatory response is critical for our survival; its absence is a death sentence. When the immune system acts in a balanced way, the process is self-limited and largely beneficial. Sometimes there is a loss of regulatory control that can result from a wide range of triggers and imbalances, in which case the process becomes chronic and destructive to the host; for example, in rheumatoid arthritis, eczema, inflammatory bowel disease, hypertension, and many other chronic diseases.

There are two basic types of immunity. The first is called "innate immunity," in which sentinel agents, primarily responsible for identifying infections or injurious substances, are widely distributed throughout the mucosal surfaces, connective tissues, and organs. The second system is called "acquired immunity" and its task is to provide an expandable army that can recognize pathogens missed by the innate system. A critical task is to be able to distinguish between self and non-self antigens. If this goes awry, they can attack the host and result in autoimmune disease. Initially, it was thought that the innate system was involved with acute inflammation, while acquired immunity resulted in chronic inflammation. However, we now recognize that a dysfunctional innate system acting in concert with vascular, metabolic, hormonal, and connective tissues plays a prominent role in instigating and perpetuating chronic inflammation. Most of this chronic inflammation is below the pain threshold, hence the name "silent inflammation." This insidious process, as we have seen, goes on year after year, largely unrecognized by both doctor and patient.

Our Modern Diet

The major cause of silent inflammation is the result of the changes that have occurred in our food supply over the past fifty years. A 1986 *New England Journal of Medicine* article by Dr. Boyd Eaton showed that the neo-Paleolithic diet of our ancestors consisted of moderate carbohydrates, moderate fats, and moderate proteins. This macronutrient composition appears to trigger an ideal hormonal response in our bodies. Our genes have changed very little in the past 2 million years and we are still ideally suited to this type of diet.

Eicosanoids, glucagon, insulin, and cortisol are the major hormones that are affected by our metabolic response to food. Eicosanoids evolved as one of the first hormonal-control systems to enable living organisms to interact with their environment. They are powerful biological agents that include leukotrienes, lipoxins, prostaglandins, and thromboxanes, all of which act on inflammation and blood flow. Research has shown that eiconsanoids provide a uni-

THE ACTIONS OF EICOSANOIDS	
GOOD EICOSANOIDS (EPA)	BAD EICOSANOIDS (ARACHIDONIC ACID)
Act as anti-inflammatories	Act as pro-inflammatories
Decrease pain transmission	Increase pain transmission
Inhibit cellular proliferation	Promote cellular proliferation
Inhibit platelet aggregation	Promote platelet aggregation
Promote vasodilation	Promote vasoconstriction
Stimulate immune response	Depress immune response

versal link to virtually every major disease, including arthritis, cancer, and heart disease.[27] Dietary fat is the only source of essential
fatty acids that form the building blocks for all eicosanoids, so it
becomes clear that some fats are indeed essential in the diet for our
well-being. Ultimately, at the molecular level, chronic disease can be
viewed as the body simply making more bad eicosanoids and fewer
good ones.

Fish, lean meats, nuts, fruits, and vegetables are part of a menu
that's in harmony with our genetic makeup, which has not changed
substantially for millenia. Our ancestors only ate from two food
groups, "meat and fish" and "vegetables and fruits." Grains only
appeared about 10,000 years ago in the Nile Valley and animal hus-
bandry started even more recently, about 7,000 years ago. A major
reason for our current epidemic of silent inflammation is our genes,
what Dr. Eaton calls "genetic discordance"—our genes have not had
time to adjust to our current lifestyle.

If you think of our ancestors just 200,000 years ago, lack of food
and potential infection with microbes and parasites were their major
threats. Our genes evolved two important mechanisms to handle
these threats. First, evolution favored those of us who were better
able to store fat to help us survive in lean times. Insulin is the
hormone that allows us to store fat, either when eating too many

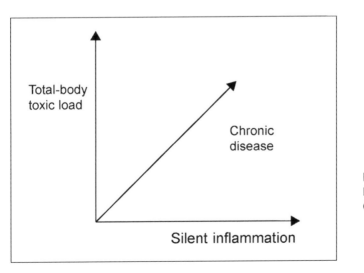

calories or too many carbohydrates. Today, we are surrounded by fast-food restaurants and stores packed with processed foods, with the result that our previous "smart genes" have not had a chance to adapt and are now killing us, as evidenced by our obesity and diabetes epidemics.

Increased insulin levels also increase the production of arachidonic acid, the building block for all pro-inflammatory eicosanoids, the major cause of silent inflammation. When our bodies are in a constant state of inflammation, our adrenal glands produce cortisol, the body's primary anti-inflammatory hormone. If silent inflammation continues, the body will be subjected to chronic elevated levels of cortisol, which results in even more obesity because cortisol increases insulin resistance. Cortisol also depresses the immune system and is known to kill brain cells and contribute to Alzheimer's disease.

Second, those of our ancestors who had an overactive immune system had a better chance of surviving pathogenic microbes. We no longer need this intense inflammatory response due to the many hygienic and social developments that ensure we have clean water and food today. Again, our genes have not had time to downregulate our inherited overactive inflammatory responses.

Returning to the Anti-Inflammatory Paleolithic Diet

By using food, you can manipulate the hormones of the body to achieve a state of optimal health, physical performance, and mental alertness. If you can change what you eat at each meal, you can be far less concerned about how much you eat. In other words, weight loss has more to do with balancing your protein, carbohydrates, and fats in the proper ratios than with your willpower. Please recognize that this is not a diet prescribed to you by a doctor or a government agency, but rather one derived from millions of years of evolutionary wisdom.

Most diet advice has been wrong because most experts do not understand how body fat is influenced by the macronutrient content of the food we eat. For example, a high-carbohydrate intake will increase your insulin levels. High insulin levels increase the levels of stored fat. We now know that the conventional wisdom of the past forty years—including the U.S. Department of Agriculture's original (now defunct) food pyramid—has been misguided.

One of the best indications that you are making too much insulin is if you are overweight and shaped like an apple. Recent research indicates that waist size may be a quick, simple, and effective predictor of heart disease risk because it measures intra-abdominal fat, the most dangerous kind of body fat.[28] For men, a waistline over forty inches indicates increased risk; for women, it's a thirty-five-inch waistline. This abdominal fat acts like an endocrine gland, with its fat cells releasing a host of pro-inflammatory toxins.

The diet of our Paleolithic ancestors—a moderate protein, carbohydrate, and fat diet—is an anti-inflammatory diet that is designed to reduce body weight, slow aging, and reverse chronic disease. Boyd

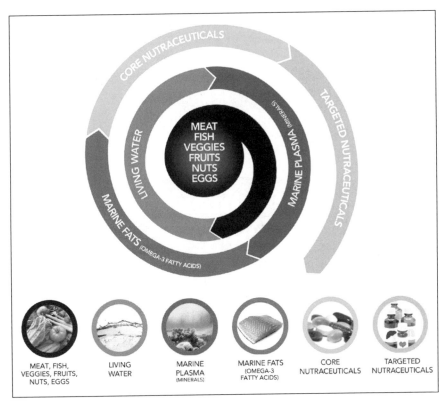

The Paleo Diet

Eaton, John Speth, and Loren Cordain estimate that Paleolithic diets were high in protein (19–35 percent) and fat (28–58 percent) and relatively low in carbohydrates (22–40 percent).[29]

The most powerful drug you can consume is the food you eat each day. Depending on the ratio and quality of macronutrients (carbohydrates, fats, proteins) you take in at each meal, your daily diet will either keep you in an optimum zone for good health or it won't. The key is to create a physiological state in which the hormones (especially insulin) influenced by the diet are kept in ranges consistent with optimal health. The Paleo Diet is an anabolic diet!

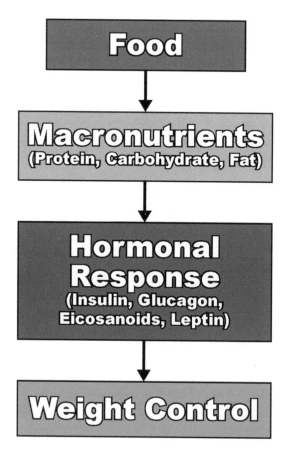

Food Is Your Most Important "Medicine"

The goal is to keep insulin levels less than 5 mU/ml. We now know that this diet helps keep eicosanoids, insulin, and weight at ideal levels, which, in turn, lowers silent inflammation levels. And remember that the health consequences of failing to keep insulin levels in range can be heart disease, insulin resistance, obesity, type 2 diabetes, and many other unwanted health complications. A large percentage of the American population has some insulin resistance.

A Balanced Immune System

Finally, an interesting observation shows an unusual link between inflammation and the environment in which you are raised. The "hygiene hypothesis" suggests that an infant's immature immune system requires a certain level of inoculation by dietary and other antigens to become fully competent. One reason for the rising incidence of allergic syndromes, inflammatory bowel disease, and auto-immune diseases (type 1 diabetes and multiple sclerosis) in modern societies could be the lack of exposure to sensitizing amounts of antigens in the first year of life. Numerous studies show that children who are raised on farms, have multiple siblings, spend time in day care, or live with cats and dogs in the first 6–12 months of life are less likely to develop allergies and other immune disorders than children from relatively sterile environments.

One of the predominant factors in determining the overall health of the individual is whether a person's immune system is operating in a balanced or unbalanced fashion. When the immune system is active in a balanced and appropriate way, the vast majority of inflammatory reactions do not create significant disturbances in a person's overall health. These reactions are adaptive in the sense that they are part of a self-regulating loop. Complex systems like the human body are, however, prone to acting in unpredictable ways. The well-known "butterfly effect" suggests that, in the right context, a butterfly (trigger) flapping its wings in New York could set off a series of events that result in a tornado in some other part of the world. In other words, when the right trigger is applied, this tiny shift in initial conditions leads to a disturbance in the overall balance of the system that results in a series of interconnected, self-amplifying, exponentially expanding reactions that become dramatically more powerful than the original shift in energy. This concept is the essence of chaos theory and provides a framework for chronic inflammation and the chronic disease it produces.

For example, NF-κB-mediated gene activation is the final common pathway for inflammatory responses. It appears to be up-regulated

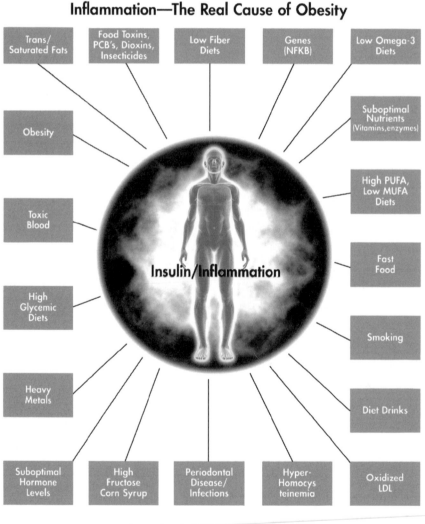

The Major Causes of Inflammation

in almost every case of acute and chronic inflammation. NF-κB (nuclear factor kappa-light-chain-enhancer of activated B cells) is a protein transcription factor found in almost all cell types and is involved in cellular responses to stimuli. NF-κB proteins can be activated by a variety of triggers, including reactive oxygen species (particularly oxidized fats), homocysteine, gliadins, lead and iron, infections, hormones, and stress.

It is also true, however, that a relatively minor intervention can sometimes create a positive perturbation that leads to homeostasis and balance once more. For example, a probiotic (friendly bacteria) supplement can cause a major change in gut flora, resulting in a series of physiological events that ultimately decreases a person's systemic allergic symptoms or migraine headaches or a chronic skin rash like eczema.

Another current example is the use of statin drugs to prevent cardiovascular disease. We now know that cardiovascular disease is a chronic inflammatory condition not due to high cholesterol, which is what statins were designed for. Statins are now becoming known for their anti-inflammatory action rather than their cholesterol-lowering effect. From a public health standpoint, it would be much more cost effective to design a diet rich in anti-inflammatory phytochemicals and low in inflammatory triggers such as trans-fats and refined carbohydrates. This can be done by functional medicine physicians who take a patient-centered approach for each specific disease rather than a dogmatic, standardized treatment. The therapeutic armamentarium is much larger and more flexible, and a rich and more colorful picture of the person's life emerges.

Acute inflammation is the body's normal response to injury or invasion by pathogens. Chronic inflammation is a maladaptive immune process responsible for a wide variety of seemingly disparate diseases. A much wider view of a person's life is needed if we are to understand the genesis of chronic inflammation:

- Dietary factors, especially refined carbohydrates, are the single most important underlying cause of silent inflammation.

- Genetic influences may predispose a person to inflammation and immune dysregulation (genes load the gun but lifestyle pulls the trigger).

- Acute or recurrent triggers can be a result of all four quadrants that may activate chronic inflammation.

- Endogenous mediators that are over-expressed in response to the triggers fuel the fire and perpetuate the chronic inflammation.

The most direct and practical way to restore homeostasis is to make dietary and lifestyle changes that will help reduce the harmful inflammatory triggers; employ a combination of antioxidants, biological response modifiers, and select therapeutic nutrients (enzymes, prebiotics, probiotics, fish oil) to assist the immune system in regaining balance; and add herbs and supplements such as ginger, boswellia, white willow bark, and bioflavonoids.

ARE YOU INFLAMED?

In reality, those who repudiate a theory that they had once proposed, or a theory that they had accepted enthusiastically and with which they had identified themselves, are very rare. The great majority of them shut their ears so as not to hear the crying facts, and shut their eyes so as not to see the glaring facts, in order to remain faithful to their theories in spite of all and everything.

—MAURICE ARTHUS,
PHILOSOPHY OF SCIENTIFIC INVESTIGATION (1921)

It is time to re-examine the true cause of our chronic diseases of civilization. I believe that "silent inflammation," caused principally by the metabolic effects resulting from a diet rich in refined carbohydrates, is the problem. We need to first diagnose inflammation and then eradicate it. We need to observe and find the underlying principles responsible for our epidemic of chronic disease.

Chronic inflammatory conditions usually reference the body site plus the suffix "-itis." These include arthritis, dermatitis, tendonitis, gastritis, bursitis, colitis, hepatitis, periodontitis, phlebitis, and bronchitis. We now know that if you have heart disease, cancer, Alzheimer's, multiple sclerosis, lupus, obesity, or any chronic disease, you have inflammation.

Silent inflammation means that you may not have an obvious pain condition or any existing chronic disease, as listed above, but that you have an insidious, ongoing disturbance of the endothelial lining of your entire cardiovascular system that is "silently" eroding your health. Until recently, there was no way to test for this. Now you can and what's more, you can make lifestyle changes that dramatically decrease silent inflammation. There are some simple dietary changes and additional select nutraceuticals that can control silent inflammation within a few weeks.

Silent Inflammation Profile (SIP)

Since eicosanoids don't circulate in the bloodstream, you cannot measure them directly. However, you can measure the key building blocks for eicosanoids in the bloodstream. The chief building block for the pro-inflammatory eicosanoids is arachidonic acid (AA); the chief building block for the anti-inflammatory eicosanoids is eicosapentaenoic acid (EPA). The AA/EPA ratio in the blood is considered by many as the gold standard test for silent inflammation. An ideal SIP ratio is 1.5. The Japanese have an average level of 1.5 and have one of the longest life spans with the lowest incidence of heart disease and depression. The average SIP for Americans is 12 and we are amongst the fattest (and most inflamed) people in the world.

Take the simple questionnaire on the following page to see if you have inflammation. Mark each statement "yes" if it applies to you, "no" if it does not.

The Lyon Diet Heart Study demonstrates the validity of the SIP. In this study, two random groups who had recently survived heart attacks were put on different diets. One followed the standard American Heart Association (AHA) diet, rich in grains and starches and

QUESTIONNAIRE: ARE YOU INFLAMED?

	YES	NO
I have plenty of energy.		
After a meal I am not hungry for 4–6 hours.		
I feel rested on waking.		
I find it easy to focus.		
My stool is usually loose or floats.		
My hair and nails are strong.		
I feel I always get enough sleep.		
I don't usually crave carbohydrates.		
I do not get headaches.		
I am not overweight.		
TOTAL:		

Scoring: If you answered "no" to three or more of the questions, you probably have a degree of silent inflammation.

high in omega-6 fatty acids (vegetable oils). The other group ate a diet rich in fruits and vegetables and low in omega-6s. After four years, the group that had reduced their omega-6s had a 70 percent reduction in fatal heart attacks. They also experienced no sudden cardiac deaths. Researchers were surprised to find no differences in cholesterol, triglycerides, glucose, or blood pressure in the two groups. The only difference was that the group with the low omega-6s had a 30 percent drop in their SIP.[30]

Fasting Insulin Levels

Just like the SIP, a fasting insulin level is also a better predictor of future risk of heart disease than cholesterol level. The higher your insulin level, the more inflammation your body is producing, because insulin causes the production of AA from omega-6s. If your fasting insulin is greater than 10 mU/ml, your chance of developing heart disease increases five times.[31] By the time your level reaches 15 mU/ml, chances are you are overweight, insulin resistant, and at risk for type 2 diabetes mellitus.

Triglyceride/High-Density Lipoprotein (HDL) Ratio

The higher your TG/HDL ratio, the higher your insulin levels and the greater the amount of silent inflammation. A level of 2 is good and less than 1 is ideal. A ratio greater than 2 identifies you as having increased silent inflammation. The average American has a TG/HDL ratio of 3.3. Those with a ratio of 4 or more are at risk for type 2 diabetes mellitus.

C-Reactive Protein (CRP)

CRP is synthesized by the liver in response to inflammation. It is a non-specific marker for inflammation. The newer high-sensitivity CRP (hs-CRP) test is more sensitive. A CRP level of 2 is good and less than 1 is ideal. Your risk of heart disease increases markedly once levels are higher than 3 mg/L. Increased fiber intake and Wobenzym significantly lower CRP. Weight loss of just 5–10 percent is associated with a dramatic reduction in inflammatory markers.

Percent Body Fat

As the percent of body fat increases, the amount of silent inflammation usually also increases. It is an easy screening test, as is the measurement of the waistline. Both of these parameters are used in diagnosing metabolic syndrome. Simply jump naked in front of a mirror and use a tape measure at the belly button—you will have a good idea if you have excess body fat and are thus inflamed.

		GOOD	IDEAL
Percent Body Fat	Male	20%	15%
	Female	25%	20%
Waist Circumference	Male	<40 inches	<35 inches
	Female	<35 inches	<30 inches

Other Medical Tests to Measure Inflammation

There are many blood tests currently available to measure silent inflammation and endothelial dysfunction. These tests are increasing in number as the critical role of inflammation is beginning to be understood

SUMMARY

- "Silent inflammation" is now recognized as the underlying cause of most chronic diseases, such as heart disease, cancer, and Alzheimer's disease, and even of aging itself.

- "We are as old as our arteries." More than 80 percent of humans die of vascular disease. Therefore, to reverse chronic disease and slow aging, we need to control "silent inflammation" in the endothelium.

- The epidemic of obesity and silent inflammation is the single biggest factor responsible for our current health-care crisis.

- Silent inflammation attacks the single layer of cells (the endothelium) that lines the many miles of blood vessels within each of us.

- The major cause of silent inflammation is the result of changes that have occurred in our food supply over the past fifty years.

- Silent inflammation can now be diagnosed with a few simple, inexpensive blood tests.

- The most powerful "drug" you can take is the food that you eat each day. The ratio of the macronutrients—carbohydrates, fats, and proteins—determines how inflamed you are. Insulin makes you fat and keeps you fat; it is only released in response to carbohydrates in your diet. A low-carbohydrate diet and omega-3 fish oil supplements are the most effective way of alleviating inflammation.

The remaining chapters will show you how to optimize your health by controlling silent inflammation.

CHAPTER 2

Nutrition

If you eat the typical North American (or Western) diet, with abundant convenience and fast foods, you likely consume an unbalanced intake of the nutrients that promote inflammation. This imbalance results in large part from the massive changes in our food supply over the past half century or so. During this time highly processed pro-inflammatory foods have largely replaced anti-inflammatory fresh and natural foods. The consequence has primed our bodies for chronic, excessive, and self-destructive levels of inflammation.
—JACK CHALLEM, *THE INFLAMMATION SYNDROME*

IN *THE PHYSIOLOGY OF TASTE,* an 1825 discourse considered among the most famous books ever written about food, French gastronome Jean Anthelme Brillat-Savarin (1755–1826) said that he could easily identify causes of obesity after thirty years of listening to one "stout party" after another proclaiming the joys of bread, rice, and potatoes. Humans never evolved to eat a diet high in starches and sugars. Grain products and concentrated sugars were essentially absent from human nutrition until the advent of agriculture just 10,000 years ago. High-calorie, carbohydrate meals rich in processed, easily digestible food and drinks can lead to an exaggerated post-prandial elevation in blood glucose and triglycerides, triggering a biochemical cascade that results in inflammation.

Close to 70 percent of the U.S. population is now overweight. Being overweight is the number one risk factor for developing diabetes, metabolic syndrome and many other chronic diseases. The good news is that we are in the middle of a medical revolution: science has unearthed how "silent inflammation" causes obesity. This dramatic breakthrough can help fix not only the rampant obesity epidemic but can help stop, and in many cases actually reverse, chronic disease.

Cardiovascular disease still remains the number one cause of death, accounting for over 40 percent of all fatalities. Without controlling inflammation, the prevalence of heart disease in the U.S. is projected to double during the next fifty years. It was American scientist Ancel Keys (1904–2004), the creator of the K-rations used by combat soldiers in the Second World War, who had an epiphany about the cause of heart disease while at a medical conference in Rome. A physiologist from Naples, Italy, claimed that heart disease was not a problem in his city. Keys found that indeed the general population of Naples was heart disease free, but the rich were not. Rich people had more heart disease than the poor, he postulated, because they ate more fat. (What Keys did not appreciate was that as the intake of meat and saturated fat increased, grain consumption decreased, but there was a dramatic increase in refined carbohydrates, white rice, flour, and sugar.)

Over the next decade, Keys gathered evidence to back his hypothesis, including his famous "Seven Countries Study." However, when all twenty-two countries he studied were included in the analysis, the apparent link between fat and heart disease vanished (but there was a very strong correlation between sugar consumption and heart disease). Interestingly, residents of the Greek islands of Corfu and Crete (two of the seven countries) consumed less than 16 pounds of sugar, honey, pastries, and ice cream per year. These countries were later to form the basis of the so-called Mediterranean diet and their inhabitants shown to have little or no heart disease.

In order to control inflammation (and our weight), it is important to understand how the science of nutrition has evolved, especially over the past 150 years. By understanding the past, we can make sense of the often conflicting nutritional views today and, more importantly, we can learn how to best control inflammation with evidence-based dietary guidelines that will allow men to finally drop those extra pounds, so that they can reverse chronic disease and slow the aging process.

THE EVOLUTION OF NUTRITION

My late friend, Hugh Riordan, M.D., nutrition expert and author of *Medical Mavericks*, summarized the evolution of nutrition into four epochs this way:

- Paleolithic Diet—Highly diverse diet, consisting of lean meats, fish, and vegetable matter. Balanced intake (1:1 ratio) of pro- and anti-inflammatory fats and very high intake of anti-inflammatory vitamins and minerals.

- Agricultural Revolution—Greatly increased intake of grains, lower intake of vegetables and meat. Displacement of nutrient-dense vegetables and meat with moderate shift toward pro-inflammatory diet.

- Industrial Revolution—Extensive refining and processing of grains and sugar, enabling large segments of the population to afford and consume such foods. Further displacement of nutrient-dense foods and great risk of elevated pro-inflammatory blood sugar levels

- Convenience/Fast-Food Revolution—Refining, processing, and industrial manipulation of foods widespread, creating a typical diet high in carbohydrates, unbalanced fat intake, and very low intake of vegetables. Diet contains 20–30 times more pro-inflammatory than anti-inflammatory fats and substantially fewer anti-inflammatory vitamins and minerals.

In 1863, William Banting (1797–1878), a retired undertaker in London, published "A Letter on Corpulence, Addressed to the Public," which launched the first popular diet craze. Within a year, *Banting* had entered the English language as a verb meaning "to diet." Banting weighed over 200 pounds and stood at 5 feet, 5 inches tall. He had consulted more than twenty of the better doctors of the day and found no help in losing weight. Finally, Banting met William Harvey, M.D., who placed Banting on a diet. Dr. Harvey had recently heard a lecture on diabetes in Paris and treated Banting successfully with animal food and vegetables that contained neither sugar nor starch (in particular, bread, milk, beer, sweets, potatoes, and pies). Despite continual ingestion of several glasses of wine and brandy daily, Banting lost over fifty pounds without any problem over the following months. For over 100 years, many physicians successfully treated patients with this low-carbohydrate diet of animal food and vegetables.

In 1961, Ancel Keys appeared on *Time* Magazine and the American Heart Association (AHA) officially alerted the nation to the dangers of dietary fat. In fact, it was Keys who deserves most of the credit for convincing us that levels of cholesterol best predict heart disease and that dietary fat is a killer. In 1957, the AHA had opposed Keys' diet/heart hypothesis. Less than four years later, although the evidence hadn't changed, a committee (which included Keys) issued a new statement, just two pages long with no references, linking elevated cholesterol to the risk of heart disease. Keys believed that the ideal heart-healthy diet should increase the percentage of carbohydrates from less than 50 percent to 70 percent and reduce fat from 40 percent to 15 percent. Our Paleolithic ancestors, by comparison, ate a diet of moderate carbohydrates (one-third), moderate fat (one-third), and moderate protein (one-third).

In 1977, Keys' hypothesis became gospel when Senator George McGovern announced the first Dietary Goals of the United States, the first time that any government institution had told Americans they could improve their health by eating less fat. Interestingly, McGovern's committee was due to be downsized to a subcommittee, which led the then staff director, Marsha Matz, to say, "We really were totally naïve, a bunch of kids who just thought, 'Hell, we should say something on this subject before we go out of business'."

There was little or no evidence to support these dietary goals. The National Institutes of Health had committed its heart disease budget to two ongoing studies. For example, the Mr. Fit Trial (1982) and the Lipid Research Clinic Trial (1984) both found no association between fat and heart disease.[1] Researchers reviewed twenty-six years of the Framingham Heart Study data and showed a significant overlap of low-density lipoprotein (LDL) cholesterol in populations with and without coronary heart disease: 80 percent of myocardial infarction patients had similar cholesterol levels as those who did not have myocardial infarctions. In addition, twice as many individuals who had a lifetime total cholesterol of less than 200 mg/dL had coronary heart disease compared to those who had a total cholesterol greater than 300 mg/dL.[2]

In contrast, a wealth of epidemiological studies showed that when populations around the world were exposed to Western diets (sugar, molasses, white flour, white rice), this caused an increase in "diseases of civilization"—obesity, diabetes, coronary heart disease, hypertension, cerebral vascular disease, cancer, diverticulitis, and gallstones, among others—all due to the increase in easily digestible carbohydrates.

Refined Carbohydrates

The refining of carbohydrates represents the biggest change in nutrition since the introduction of agriculture 10,000 years ago. Unfortunately, the link between refined carbohydrates and disease had been obscured over the years by the insufficient appreciation of the correlation between carbohydrates in the natural state and the unnatural refined carbohydrates; that is, treating sugars and white flour as equivalent to raw fruits, vegetables, and whole-meal flour.

Earlier researchers had measured only fat, protein, and total carbohydrates, thus failing to account for the effects of these refined carbohydrates. In fact, in Keys' Seven Countries Study, sugar consumption predicted coronary artery disease far more than saturated fats. Others also showed that increased sugar consumption (increased insulin and triglycerides) correlates better than cholesterol with coronary artery disease.[3] Prominent researchers in the 1920s refused to believe that carbohydrates caused diabetes, which unknowingly led four decades of endocrinologists to believe that increased fat was the causative factor in diabetes.[4]

In the 1960s, Robert Stout suggested that the ingestion of large quantities of refined carbohydrates leads to hyperinsulinemia and insulin resistance, and then to atherosclerosis and heart disease.[5] In certain individuals, insulin secretion, after eating carbohydrates, can be disproportionately large, with carbohydrates being disposed of in fat tissues, the liver, and arterial walls. This ultimately leads to obesity. Anything that raises blood sugar, especially refined carbohydrates, will generate free radicals, increasing the rate of oxidative stress and the formation of advanced glycation end products (AGEs). This will lead to more atherosclerosis and vascular disease, with an accelerated pace of physical degeneration, even in those who never actually become diabetic.

In the mid-1970s, Gerald Reaven, a researcher at Stanford University, in Palo Alto, California, initiated the study of the glycemic index to test the difference between simple and complex carbohydrates. Dr. Reaven was more interested in insulin and left this research to David Jenkins and others. In the 1980s, Dr. Reaven

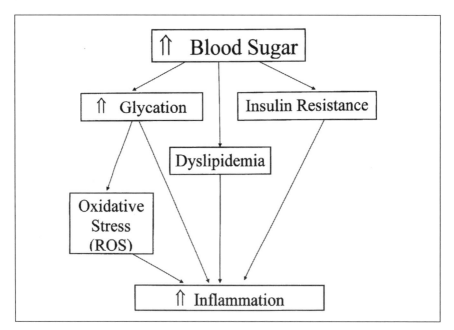

Importance of Avoiding Elevated Blood Sugars

coined the term *Syndrome X* (also known as metabolic syndrome or insulin resistance syndrome) to describe the metabolic abnormalities in obesity (diabetes and cardiovascular disease), all exacerbated by sugar, flour, and other easily digestible carbohydrates. Insulin resistance syndrome consists of:

* Increased triglycerides and LDL cholesterol (the "bad" kind)

* Decreased high-density lipoprotein (HDL) cholesterol (the "good" kind)

* Increased fibrinogen and C-reactive protein (inflammatory markers)

* Increased uric acid

* Increased blood sugar and insulin

* Increased waist size (obesity)

* Increased blood pressure

Insulin is the primary regulator of fat, carbohydrate, and protein metabolism. Species need time to adapt fully to changes in the environment—the introduction of diets high in sugar and refined, easily digestible carbohydrates was the most dramatic change to the body over the past 2 million years. **It is probable that refined carbohydrates and sugar created such a disturbance in blood glucose and insulin that they led to a profound disturbance of homeostatic regulation and growth throughout the entire body.**

Physician William Osler noted in 1882 at Johns Hopkins Hospital that only 10 out of 35,000 patients were diagnosed with diabetes mellitus. Diabetes today is at epidemic proportions: over 1 million new cases will be diagnosed this year. Eternity Medicine Institute and Heart Check America now inexpensively screen for heart disease and its metabolic causes such as diabetes, obesity, and metabolic syndome.

In 1978, high-fructose corn syrup (HFCS) was introduced into the U.S. market, containing 55 percent fructose and 45 percent glucose, identical with sucrose (table sugar). By 1985, one-half of all sugar consumed in the U.S. was from corn sweeteners and two-thirds of this was HFCS. This was initially perceived as healthy because fructose appeared not to increase blood sugar because it had a low glycemic index. The problem was there was a dramatic increase in triglycerides by the liver and increased storage of fat—fructose-induced lipogenesis. Fructose is, in fact, the most lipogenic carbohydrate and it increases blood pressure much more than sucrose. In addition, fructose produces ten times more X-linking of proteins. Once proteins are X-linked, they are unable to perform properly in the body; people who are obese or have diabetes have two to three times the number of X-linked proteins. Thus, HFCS is the worst of both worlds—glucose increases insulin and fructose increases triglycerides. I believe that the reason the U.S. population went from being 15 percent overweight in 1985 to 70 percent today is primarily due to the HFCS.

The excessive consumption of these refined carbohydrates leads to obesity and diabetes. This excess weight and obesity are caused by the singular hormonal effects of a diet rich in refined and easily digestible carbohydrates. It is the "quality" of these calories consumed that regulates weight and the "quantity" (more calories consumed than expended) that is a secondary phenomenon. There is something about carbohydrates that allows an increased consump-

MODERN FOODS AND THEIR CALORIES PER POUND

Food	Calories/Pound
Salad	100
Fruit	300
Potato, rice, beans	500
Ice cream	1,200
Bread	1,500
Sugar	1,800
Chocolate	2,500
Oils	4,000

tion of food but still induces hunger. This is because the flow of fatty acids out of the cells and into the circulation depends on the level of blood sugar and insulin levels. If sugar and insulin levels are high in the blood, then free fatty acids cannot be released from the cells. At a cellular level the body is in fact starving, and this manifests as continual hunger and lethargy.

Despite our modern understanding of the role of high-glycemic carbohydrates in producing inflammation and most chronic disease, it is amazing how the cholesterol hypothesis of heart disease refuses to go away. Even though many now acknowledge that metabolic syndrome (now estimated to affect 60 percent of adults over the age of sixty) is probably the cause of most heart disease in America, and that this syndrome is likely caused by the excessive consumption of refined carbohydrates, many remain wedded to the cholesterol/heart disease dogma.

THE GLYCEMIC INDEX

When researchers tested different foods, they found that some simple sugars entered the bloodstream very slowly, whereas some complex carbohydrates like potatoes entered the bloodstream faster than table sugar. Every complex carbohydrate must be broken down into simple sugars and will eventually enter the bloodstream as glucose, which in turn will stimulate insulin. Fiber (both soluble and insoluble) cannot be broken down into simple sugars and thus will have no effect on insulin. If a carbohydrate source like pasta, which has little fiber, is tested, there is a high insulin response as compared with broccoli, which is rich in fiber, where the insulin response will be minimal. This is why starches and grains are considered high-density carbohydrates, fruits are medium density, and vegetables are low density.

The glycemic index (GI) is a measure of the entry rates of various carbohydrate sources into the bloodstream. The faster their rate of entry, the greater the effect on insulin secretion, and the higher the GI score. There are at least five factors that affect the glycemic index of a particular carbohydrate:

- The physical state of the starch in a food is the most important factor influencing glycemic index (the less gelatinized [swollen] the starch, the slower the rate of digestion).

- The amount of fiber, especially soluble fiber.

- The amount of fat—this slows the rate of stomach emptying, which slows the digestion of starch.

- Composition of the complex carbohydrate—the digestion of sugar produces only half as many glucose molecules as the same amount of starch.

- The acidity of foods—acids in foods slow emptying and digestion.

The glycemic load (GL) is even more important than the glycemic index in determining the insulin output of a meal. The glycemic load is the actual amount of insulin-stimulating carbohydrates consumed multiplied by its glycemic index.

GLYCEMIC IMPACT OF DIFFERENT FOODS			
SOURCE	VOLUME	GLYCEMIC INDEX (GI)	GLYCEMIC LOAD (GL)
Pasta	1 cup	59	3,068
Apple	1 cup	54	972
Broccoli	1 cup	50	150

Note: For further examples, see *The New Glucose Revolution* by Jennie Brand-Miller, Thomas Wolever, Kaye Foster-Powell, and Stephen Colaqiuri (New York: Marlowe & Company, 2002).

Even though the GI of each of these carbohydrates is about the same, 1 cup of pasta generates twenty times the insulin response of 1 cup of broccoli. Remember, the more processed a food, the higher the GL. Thus, by using the concept of glycemic load, it also becomes clear why consuming most of your carbohydrates from quality vegetables and fruits is key to maintaining low insulin levels.

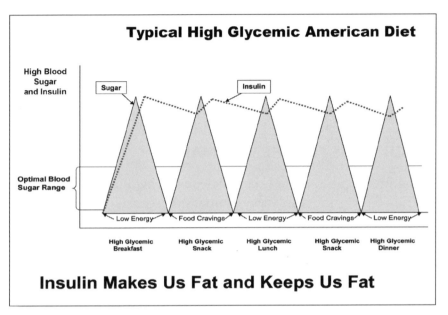

Typical High-Glycemic American Diet and High Insulin Levels

As the glycemic index and glycemic load of your diet increases, so do hunger, cravings, binge eating, and overeating. They are promoted by high-glycemic foods. On the other hand, if you switch to a low-glycemic diet, your insulin levels will fall and enable fatty acids to be released by your cells, which will produce fewer cravings and allow you to lose weight. Here are a number of ways to do this:

- Use breakfast cereals based on oats, barley, bran, fiber, and lack of sugar

- Use "grainy" breads made with whole seeds (3 to 5 grams of fiber per slice)

- Reduce the amount of potatoes you eat—substitute with yams

- Enjoy most types of fruits and vegetables

- Eat plenty of salads with vinaigrette dressing

- Avoid sugar and sugar products

- Eat 4–6 small meals daily

- Eat healthy fat and protein with your carbohydrates

- Eat fiber with your carbohydrates

- Eat slowly

WEIGHT LOSS FOR THE WELLMAN

When investigators tested the efficiency of high-fat, carbohydrate-restricted diets, the results were remarkably constant. Every investigator reported weight loss of 1–5 pounds per week. None suffered symptoms of semi-starvation or food deprivation, excessive fatigue, irritability, mental depression, or extreme hunger.[6]

If we add 400 calories of fat and protein to 800 calories of protein and fat, we have a 1,200 calorie high-fat, carbohydrate-restricted diet that will result in considerable weight loss, but if we add 400 calories of carbohydrates to 800 calories of protein and fat, we have a balanced semi-starvation diet usually prescribed for obesity. We now have a diet that will induce 40 pounds of weight loss in less than 1 in 100 instead of 1 in 2. This means that if you just reach for a bagel or a couple of sodas, you would now be eating a balanced semi-starvation diet with its 1 percent success rate.

In the 1920s, New York internist Blake Donaldson treated over 17,000 patients with a low-carbohydrate diet with good success. Alfred Pennington, M.D., followed Donaldson with excellent results.[7] The diet consisted of a half-pound of fatty meat three times a day with a "hotel portion" of raw fruit or a potato to substitute for the roots and berries of prehistoric man. However, the *Journal of the American Medical Association* did not endorse such a high-protein/high-fat, low-carbohydrate diet from this time until 2004, despite the numerous clinical studies presented over the years.

There is a wealth of conflicting diet advice out there today. Not surprisingly, most of us remain confused about this subject and often still buy into one or more of the prevailing myths about weight gain and weight loss.

EIGHT MYTHS ABOUT WEIGHT GAIN

1. The #1 Dietary Myth—Eat less + exercise more = weight loss.

2. The Starvation Myth—Skipping meals will help weight loss.

3. The Fat Myth—Eating fat makes you fat.

4. The Caloric Myth—A calorie is a calorie.

5. The Artificial Sweetener Myth—Diet sodas (and artificial sweeteners) help you lose weight.

6. The Toxin Myth—Environmental toxins have nothing to do with weight loss.

7. The Government Protector Myth—Government knows best.

8. The Water Myth—All water is the same.

To counter these myths, I offer the eight integral keys to permanent weight loss, all of which are covered in this book.

EIGHT KEYS TO PERMANENT WEIGHT LOSS

1. Inflammation—Control inflammation (insulin makes us fat and keeps us fat).

2. Nutrition—A return to the diet of our Paleolithic ancestors will promote weight loss.

3. Toxin Reduction—Detoxifying will increase your fat burning by more than 20 percent.

4. Exercise—Increasing your exercise level is critical for weight distribution and maintenance.

5. Ground Water—Consume alkaline water only to help weight loss.

6. Restore Hormones—Optimize your hormones to optimize weight loss.

7. Advanced Supplementation—Smart supplementation can help you

reduce inflammation and oxidation, improve energy, and detoxify, all necessary for sustained weight reduction.

8. Lifelong (Mind-Body) Learning—Knowledge, relaxation, and a good night's sleep makes you thin.

THE PALEOLITHIC PRESCRIPTION

It is important first that you recognize that this is not just another diet prescribed to you by some authors, a diet center, or a government agency, but rather the "original human diet." Our genetic makeup, shaped through the millennia, determines our nutritional and activity needs. Accumulating evidence suggests that the mismatch between our modern diet and lifestyle and our Paleolithic genome is responsible for the epidemic of obesity and the diseases of civilization that now afflict us.

Until just 500 generations ago, all humans consumed only wild and unprocessed food foraged and hunted from their environment. This provided a diet high in lean proteins, polyunsaturated (omega-3s) and monounsaturated fats, fiber, vitamins, minerals, antioxidants, and other beneficial phytonutrients. The WellMan diet is designed to simulate the milieu for which we are genetically designed. Using this evolutionary wisdom, we can see how diets like Atkins and Ornish make little or no sense.

In a recent review of approximately 150 studies on the link between diet and cardiovascular health, the authors concluded that three major dietary approaches have emerged as the most effective in preventing heart disease:

• Replacing saturated and trans-fats with monounsaturated and polyunsaturated fats

• Increasing consumption of omega-3 fats from either fish or plant sources

• Eating a diet high in various fruits, vegetables, nuts, and whole grains and avoiding foods with a high-glycemic load

This report, likewise, found no relationship between cardiovascular disease and intake of meat, cholesterol, or total fat.[8]

FUNDAMENTALS OF THE PALEOLITHIC DIET AND LIFESTYLE

- Eat whole, natural, fresh foods; avoid highly processed and high-glycemic-load foods.

- Consume a diet high in fruits, vegetables, nuts, and berries and low in refined grains and sugars. Nutrient-dense, low-glycemic-load fruits and vegetables such as berries, plums, citrus, apples, cantaloupe, spinach, tomatoes, broccoli, cauliflower, and avocados are best.

- Increase consumption of omega-3 fatty acids from fish, fish oil, and plant sources.

- Avoid trans-fats entirely and limit intake of saturated fats. This means eliminating fried foods, hard margarine, commercial baked goods, and most packaged and processed snack foods. Substitute monounsaturated and polyunsaturated fats for saturated fats.

- Increase consumption of lean protein, such as skinless poultry, fish, game meats, and lean cuts of red meat. Cuts with the words *round* or *loin* in the name usually are lean. Avoid high-fat dairy and fatty, salty processed meats such as bacon, sausage, and deli meats.

- Incorporate olive oil and/or non-trans-fatty acid canola oil into the diet.

- Drink alkaline water.

- Participate in daily exercise from various activities, incorporating aerobic and strength training and stretching exercises. Outdoor activities are ideal.[9] The more varied the exercise, the better.

Fats

One of the most important findings to come out of recent research is that our bodies function most efficiently when we eat fats that con-

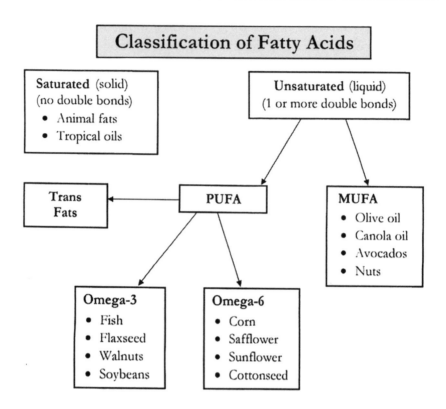

Omega-6 to Omega-3 Ratios

- Americans consume large amounts of vegetable oils that are very high in omega-6 FAs (corn, safflower, sunflower, and cottonseed)

- Americans also eat large quantities of meats from domesticated animals fed grains high in omega-6 FAs

- Our intake of omega-3 fatty acids is very low

- The ratio of omega-6 fatty acids to omega-3 FA is now greater than 20:1. (In the early human diet it was 1 to 1.)

- A ratio of 10 to 1 or higher puts us at high risk for inflammation and thrombosis—the precipitating cause of most heart attacks and strokes!

- We _**must**_ consume more omega-3 FA and less omega-6 FA!

tain a balanced ratio of the two main families of essential fatty acids, omega-6s and omega-3s. The ratio of the typical American diet has been estimated to be greater than 20:1 in favor of omega-6s. The traditional diet of the Greek island of Crete first came to the attention of the medical community in the 1960s, when Keys' study revealed that the men of Crete were healthier than 12,000 other men surveyed in seven different countries (Greece, Italy, the Netherlands, Finland, Yugoslavia, Japan, and the U.S.). Compared to the U.S., the man from Crete had half the cancer risk and only 5 percent of the mortality from coronary artery disease. The difference was due to the increased omega-3s in the diet of Crete.[10]

These findings were confirmed in the Lyon Heart Study (involving 600 patients)[11] and the Indo-Mediterranean Diet Heart Study (involving 1,000 patients).[12] When the typical low-fat American Heart Association diet was compared with the Mediterranean diet (a similar diet as our Paleolithic ancestors), which is high in omega-3s, monounsaturated fats, fruits, vegetables, and nuts, the Mediterranean diet was superior in its health benefits. Epidemiological studies show that frequent nut consumption (five or more times per week) is associated with a 50 percent reduction in risk of myocardial infarction, compared with the risk of people who never eat nuts.[13]

Americans consume large amounts of vegetable oils that are very high in omega-6 fatty acids (corn, safflower, sunflower, and cottonseed). We also eat large quantities of meats from domesticated animals fed grains high in omega-6s. Plus, our intake of omega-3 fatty acids is very low. A ratio of 10 to 1 or higher puts us at high risk for inflammation and thrombosis, the precipitating cause of most heart attacks and strokes. We *must* consume more omega-3s and less omega-6s. Increase your intake of omega-3 fatty acids from fish, krill, calamari, New Zealand mussels, or hemp.

Protein

All evidence points to the fact that hunter-gatherers were omnivores. In addition, vegetarian diets are difficult to follow and are not necessarily associated with better health.[14] A study of two groups of

Bantu villagers in Tanzania compared 618 people who lived on a lakeshore and consumed large amounts of fish to 645 people who lived in the nearby hills and were vegetarians. The lifestyle, gene pools, and diets (except for the fish) were similar in the two groups. The fish-consuming group had lower blood pressure, lower triglyceride, cholesterol, and leptin levels, and higher omega-3 levels than the vegetarian group.[15] Most vegetarian diets are often far worse, consisting of heavily processed carbohydrates such as white rice, potatoes, white flour, and sugars.

The South Asian paradox refers to the relatively high prevalence of coronary heart disease despite low levels of LDL ("bad") cholesterol and low prevalence of obesity in urban vegetarians from India who consume a diet high in refined carbohydrates.[16] Although increased meat consumption in Western diets (with increased refined carbohydrates) has been associated in some studies with increased cardiovascular disease, hunter-gatherer societies were free of the signs and symptoms of heart disease, despite being meat eaters. It may not be the amount of meat eaten but rather the composition of the meat and the cooking methods that most determine the health effects of the food. Lean animal protein eaten with each meal improves satiety levels, increases dietary thermogenesis, improves insulin sensitivity, and thus facilitates weight loss, while providing essential nutrients.

Carbohydrates

Our Paleolithic ancestors consumed a diet high in fruits, vegetables, nuts, and berries and low in refined grains and sugars (except for seasonally available honey). More than 50 percent of the carbohydrates consumed by Americans are from refined grains and are high in sugar. Most carbohydrates consumed in America are not from whole grains and are not high in dietary fiber.

Eat at least one serving per day of whole grains, such as whole-grain breads with high fiber content (3–5 grams per slice) and high-fiber cereals. "Multi-grain" or "high fiber" does not necessarily mean whole grain. Whole grains contain all three parts of the grain kernel: fiber-rich bran, the starchy endosperm, and the nutrient-packed germ. Whole grains reduce risk of cardiovascular disease, type 2 diabetes, and obesity. They can play a significant role in weight management and weight loss. Whole grains lower CRP and IL-6 levels, both markers of silent inflammation.

Grains to avoid:

- White bread

- White flour

- White rice

- High-sugar cereals (especially those with high-fructose corn syrup)

- White bagels

- White pasta

- Other white flour products

ADOPTING THE PALEOLITHIC PLAN

- Eat six small meals a day; never skip a meal

- Eat protein and healthy fats with every meal

- Eat good carbohydrates (seven servings fresh fruit/vegetables each day)

- Completely eliminate high-glycemic carbs (breads, pasta, rice, potatoes, sweets, most cereals, etc.)

- Eat 25–35 grams of fiber each day

- Drink water (at least eight to ten 8-ounce servings of alkaline water per day)

- Minimize your intake of alcohol, especially beer

- Take supplements (vitamins and minerals) each day

- Take 2.5–5.0 grams omega-3 fish oil daily

- Avoid all diet sodas and artificial sweeteners

It is important to recognize that the body does not distinguish between a soda and a diet soda. As soon as it tastes something sweet, the body will bump up its insulin level, with all its negative consequences. Studies have also shown that rats (and humans) will eat 2.5 times more food when fed diet drinks as compared with regular sweetened drinks.[17] The number of Americans who consume sugar-free, artificially sweetened products has grown from less than 70 million in 1987 to more than 160 million in 2000.[18] Artificial sweeteners may interfere with the body's natural ability to count calories based on a food's sweetness and makes people prone to overindulging in other sweet foods and beverages.[19] Research has shown that people who drink diet soda had a higher risk of developing metabolic syndrome, obesity, and heart disease.[20]

Grocery Store List

Remember, when you go shopping, shop at the periphery of the store, where most of the fresh produce is. Once you move to the center of the store, the aisles are filled with products with high-fructose corn syrup. Take care with what you put in your grocery basket—you will not eat high-glycemic foods if you don't put them in your basket to begin with. Instead, fill your basket with:

- Fruits and vegetables
- Fish (salmon, steelhead trout, tuna, and sardines)
- Olive oil and canola oil; avocados
- Omega-3 enriched eggs, free range
- Whole-grain breads (3–5 grams of fiber per slice)
- Vinaigrette salad dressing
- Chicken/turkey breasts
- High-fiber cereal
- Skim milk or almond milk

- Low-fat dairy products (white cheeses, Greek yogurts, cottage cheese)

- Yams

- Avoid legumes

SUMMARY

- Dietary fat, whether saturated or not, is not a cause of obesity, heart disease, or any other chronic disease of civilization.

- Diets high in refined carbohydrates are the chief cause for most of the chronic diseases that now afflict Americans.

- Dietary changes in our food supply over the past fifty years are the biggest cause of our health crisis.

- High intakes of refined carbohydrates cause an increase in insulin that produces "silent inflammation" and blood vessel disease (endothelial dysfunction).

- The higher the glycemic index (GI) and glycemic load (GL) of carbohydrates, the higher the insulin and inflammation in the blood vessels.

- The Paleolithic diet is the best way to reverse obesity and chronic disease.

- Not all water is the same. Alkaline water is the single most important beverage you can consume.

- Eating eggs for breakfast helps reduce calorie consumption throughout the day by 18 percent.

CHAPTER 3

Toxin Reduction

*The current level of chemicals in the food and water
supply and indoor and outdoor environment has lowered
our threshold of resistance to disease and has altered
our body's metabolism, causing enzyme dysfunction,
nutritional deficiencies, and hormonal imbalances.*
—MARSHALL MANDELL, M.D.

THE SUBJECT OF DETOXIFICATION has been absent from mainstream allopathic medicine. During the past two decades, I have watched the devastating effects of toxins on the human body and the myriad health problems they produce as the overwhelming number of chemicals we are exposed to increases our total toxic body load each day. As the toxic load increases, so does silent inflammation and the incidence of chronic diseases like obesity, heart disease, and cancer.

WHERE DO TOXINS COME FROM?

Our Paleolithic ancestors did not have toxins in their world. Unfortunately, twenty-first century humans have overrun the world with pollution, and there are no places on earth where we have not left our footprint.

By definition, a toxin is "a poisonous substance" (the word comes from the Greek *toxikon*, which means "poison"). Today, we use the word to mean anything that doesn't agree with us—a "toxic" spouse or work environment, a household or industrial pollutant, or pharmaceutical and recreational drugs (including alcohol and nicotine). Generally speaking, we can divide all toxins into two groups depending on their origin, either from external to the body (environmental toxins) or from various metabolic processes within the body (internal toxins).

Environmental Toxins

From the Air We Breathe

Industry releases, for example, the leftovers from plastic manufacturing, dioxins and polychlorinated biphenyls (PCBs), and clouds carry these potent carcinogens to every part of the globe and every body of water. They are then taken up by the soil, plants, animals, and then humans. Industry uses between 75,000 and 100,000 chemicals, with an additional 1,000 introduced each year. The Environmental Protection Agency (EPA) annually collects data on 650 of these from all fifty states. In 2005, disposal and release of just these 650 chemicals totaled nearly 43.4 billion pounds from 23,500 U.S. facilities, and nearly half of this was released via air emissions. The health effects of less than 10 percent of these chemicals have been tested. One of the concerns with toxins in the environment is that we are at the top of the food chain. When we sit down to a meal, we are exposed to the full range of chemicals and additives that have been used across the entire agricultural food chain (bioaccumulation).

Auto exhaust is another contaminant of our air. These exhausts contain heavy metals; pesticides, organic hydrocarbons (formaldehyde, benzene, and toluene), and many other chemicals, all lumped under the term *xenobiotics*. The interiors of cars are no better, as they contain high levels of polyvinyl chloride (PVC) and many other toxins.

Any chemical you can smell in the air makes its way through your lungs into the bloodstream and is then disseminated to all your organs. Air pollution kills more people worldwide each year than automobile accidents. Air pollution, as we can see, comes from

The EPA's 33 Most Hazardous Air Toxins

Acetaldehyde	Coke oven emissions	Mercury
Acrolein	1,3, Dichloropropene	Methylene chloride
Acrylonitrile	Diesel matter	Nickel
Arsenic	Ethylene dibromide	Perchlorethylene
Benzene	Ethylene dichloride	PCBs
Berrylium	Ethylene oxide	POM
Butadiene	Formaldehyde	Propylene dichloride
Cadmium	Hexachlorobenzene	Quinoline
Carbon tetrachloride	Hydrazine	Tetrachloroethylene
Chloroform	Lead	Trichloroethylene
Chromium	Manganese	Vinyl chloride

many different sources: factories, power plants, municipal incinerators, dry cleaners, cars and trucks, and even windblown dust and wildfires. Of the 188 known air toxins, the top thirty-three that the EPA considers the greatest threat to our health are found everywhere. No place is safe. Even living in the woods does not keep you safe, as the evening breezes bring you those industry and transportation emissions, which settle over you as you sleep. In fact, some suburbanites are getting worse air quality than if they lived right next door to the factories.

From the Water We Drink

As Brenda Watson writes in her excellent book *The Detox Strategy*, "The pollution and toxicity of our oceans, lakes, waterways, groundwater, and drinking water is having a devastating impact on our health and the health of our planet. . . .Water supplies must originate from somewhere, but these sources are becoming infected with pollutants from a variety of places—power plants, factories, septic systems, sewage spills, waste disposal sites for hazardous materials that sink into the groundwater, animal feed lots, landfills, acid water run off from mines, disposal wells, land disposal of sludge, spray irri-

gation, buried storage tanks and pipelines, and even from us dump-
ing things down the drain like cosmetics and unused drugs. . . . All
these water contaminants in turn affect the food we eat because they
become part of the soil and water supplies that ultimately nourish
and grow our food."[1]

In 2002, the first study of synthetic chemicals and hormones in
139 streams was undertaken and 80 percent were found to be contaminated.[2] More than a decade before, a front-page story in *USA
Today* showed that the average city water already contained over 500
different chemicals. Many of us know that the addition of fluoride (a
potent enzyme inhibitor) had little or no effect on tooth decay but
rather damaged brain enzymes and lowered IQs, in addition to other
problems it produced. Chlorine (a free radical initiator) has similarly
been shown to elevate cholesterol, accelerate aging, hasten arteriosclerosis, and increase rectal and bladder cancers.[3]

Researchers have also shown that just by showering in city water
we absorb damaging amounts of everyday chemicals like chlorine
and chloroform through our skin. The source of the water may not
be the only problem. Copper, lead, PVC, acrylates, vinylidene, and
other plastic components can leach out from pipes and conduits of
the water being transported. Interestingly, pharmaceutical chemicals
are not regulated by the EPA, so there are no enforced limits of pharmaceuticals (such as antidepressants, antibiotics, hormones, pain-
killers) in our drinking water.

From the Food We Eat

Over 90 percent of money that Americans spend on food is used to
buy processed food. This poor nutrition, together with the ever-
increasing onslaught of toxins on the body, is a recipe for disaster.
We have also to contend with a new threat—genetically modified
food. Two of the prime targets for genetic engineering, soy and corn,
may produce serious consequences, such as allergic reactions and
resistance to certain antibiotics.

A major problem with the infiltration of fast food into our modern lifestyle, besides the obesity epidemic, is that this increasing
"malnutrition" causes a host of nutritional deficiencies that directly

affect the body's ability to ward off illness from the incoming toxins. For example, in the last twenty-five years, the level of vitamin C deficiency has increased from 3 percent to 20 percent, largely due to the shift from whole foods to processed foods and fast foods. Meanwhile, U.S. agriculture uses 10 pounds of pesticide per person on the food supply each year.[4]

Sherry Rogers, M.D., in her book *Detoxify or Die*, writes, "The plastic wraps swaddling your fruits, vegetables, and meats in your grocery cart look harmless enough. So do the Styrofoam trays that hold them and the plastic bottles for water, soda, milk, ketchup, fruit juices, and even infant formula. But the phthalates that outgas from these plastics, so ubiquitous in our food and beverage packaging, leach into our foods."[5] Once these phthalates enter our bodies, they hook onto different cell parts and interfere with many metabolic processes. For example, they can damage hormone receptors and lead to loss of sex drive, they can damage brain chemistry and lead to depression and learning disorders, and they can trigger cancers of the breast, lung, prostate, and thyroid. Stealth poisons lurk in those Styrofoam coffee cups; once inside the body, there is no mechanism to get rid of all the carcinogenic styrene.

Another common food contaminant is dioxin (Agent Orange). Dioxins are made from plastics, pesticides, and other chemicals, and they are released from smoke stacks, taken up by the clouds, and rain down on our oceans and soils. Dioxin is found in fish, plants, and animals that we use for food. It is one of the most potent carcinogens known. Other pesticide-like cousins, hexachlorobenzene (HCB), PCBs, dichloro-diphenyl-trichloroethane (DDT), lindane. and atrazine all can act as synthetic hormonal look-alikes or EEDs (environmental endocrine disruptors). Non-biodegradable detergents, polystyrene, and trichloroethylene are also potent EEDs.

Bisphenol A (BPA) is another plastic and resin product used to line metal food and drink cans. It is allowed in unlimited amounts in consumer products and has been associated with infertility and breast and prostate cancers. Teflon-coated pans are no better: when heated, Teflon's chemical off-gassing can kill certain birds if they are in the same room.[6]

Food and aroma scientists manipulate volatile chemicals to create particular tastes and smells. Approximately 10,000 new processed food products are introduced each year, and the majority will require flavor additives and coloring. Infants and children are particularly sensitive to these additives and they are probably responsible for many allergies and behavioral abnormalities.

Heavy metals are another deadly toxin in our food. Cadmium, aluminum, mercury, antimony, lead, and arsenic are some of the heavy metals added to the food chain. Since the Industrial Revolution, production and distribution of heavy metals have contaminated the air, water, and topsoil of the planet. Once these toxic metals have accumulated in the body, they migrate from the blood into the tissues and are not able to be released unless they are chelated out of the body. These heavy metals disrupt metabolic processes and inhibit detoxification. They are especially toxic to the mitochondria, the energy-producing furnaces inside every cell. It is estimated that one in four Americans have heavy metal toxicity.[7]

From the Homes (and Offices) We Live In

Homes are of special significance because we spend most of our time in them. Both homes and offices have become more hazardous in recent years as we continue to "tighten" them and keep all windows closed. Health problems related to closed-up indoor environments even have their own name—sick building syndrome.

In the 1970s, many individuals unknowingly insulated their homes and offices with urea foam formaldehyde insulation (UFFI). Although UFFI was initially represented as safe, people developed brain fog, depression, headache, asthma, arthritis, and nausea; some were totally incapacitated. Formaldehyde is a known carcinogen. Carpet is known to outgas more than a dozen toxic chemicals, including benzene, toluene, xylene, butadiene, styrene, and formaldehyde. Kawasaki syndrome has been linked to gases coming off professionally cleaned carpets.

As Dr. Rogers writes, "Construction materials like paints and wallboard plasticizers in wallpaper, phenols in plywood, formaldehyde in pressed-wood kitchen cabinets, bookcases, and dresser drawers, and wood preservatives are just a few of the common construction materials, not to mention foam formaldehyde in sofas, chairs, mattresses, and boron insulation. Back drafts from creosote-lined chimneys and flues can trigger symptoms."[8] Mattresses and pillows, in addition to formaldehyde, contain pesticides and fire retardant. Wool blankets can emit trichloroethylene dry cleaning fluid and moth-deterring pesticides. Choose natural fibers such as cotton, linen, wool, and hemp. When you do dry cleaning, let the garments aerate outside for a day before putting them in your closet.

Further indoor pollutants are appliances and computers with their plastic housings, hydrocarbon glues, and formaldehyde finishings. Many of these appliances also put out damaging electromagnetic frequencies (EMFs).

Rid your house or office of any molds. They are powerful EEDs and contain lethal cancer-causing mycotoxins.

Do not use pesticides in the home. There is a higher incidence of leukemia in children due to pesticide use. Also, beware of insecticides. I remember a lawn services company spraying my neighbor's back lawn. Their new puppy, which played on the lawn for the rest of the day, was dead by the following morning. Coincidence? I think not!

The home also has other problems. The faulty furnace, the paints, solvents, oils, gas appliance—all are ever present in every household. There are also air purifiers designed for every use (smoke, chemicals, gases, fumes, molds, bacteria, and viruses), which can do more harm than good. Deodorants, soaps, detergents, toothpaste, and cosmetics may also contain harmful ingredients. The most active ingredient in deodorant is aluminum, a known toxin implicated in Alzheimer's disease (also beware of aluminum cooking pans and cans). Antibacterial soaps kill the good as well as harmful bacteria. Use natural organic detergents rather than commercial toxic ones. Beware the known toxins in cosmetics—paraben, diethanolamine (DEA), ureas, petrolatum, propylene glycol, and synthetic colors and fragrances, among others.

Although it's not practical to remodel your house or place of business, you can do a lot to reduce your environmental exposure to toxins. You can control what you bring into your environment and you can more wisely select those products that will help rather than harm your health.

Internal Toxins

The byproducts of our metabolism of proteins, carbohydrates, and fats need to be processed. Bacteria and yeast in our gut also produce waste products, metabolic products, and cellular debris that can interfere with many of our bodily functions. These products, in addition to inhaled, ingested, and absorbed foreign chemicals, go through a two-phase detoxification process in most cells in the body.

Phase I detoxification occurs in the endoplasmic reticulum of the cell. Either oxidation, reduction, or hydrolysis occurs. Often, this is all that needs to be done and the metabolite is excreted in the urine. However, if the kidneys get overloaded, a back-up system kicks in. In Phase II detoxification, a large protein or amino acid is hooked onto a metabolite, making it bigger, more electrically charged, and hence more polar. In this form, it is more soluble in water and can be more easily excreted through the bile into the stool. This is called conjugation. The glutathione pathway accounts for 60 percent of Phase II activity.

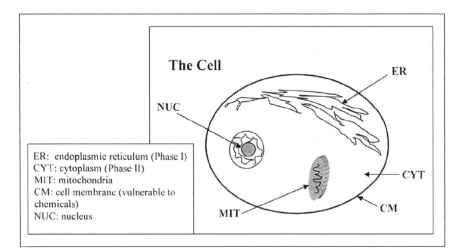

The Cell

Remember, the intestinal lining houses not only half of the immune system but also half of the detoxifying system. Many people's intestines are overloaded with bacteria like *Klebsiella* and *Citrobacter* (from poor nutrition) and yeasts like *Candida* (from excess antibiotics). These factors over time can produce a "leaky gut." The inflamed gut is damaged and abnormal spaces open up in the intestinal wall. Leakage of toxins then occurs into the bloodstream, not

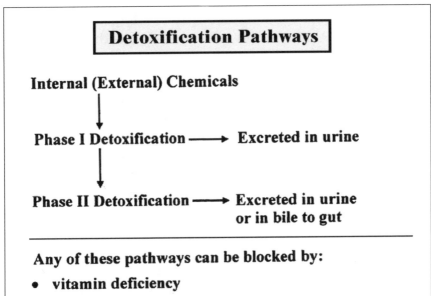

Detoxification Pathways

Internal (External) Chemicals

Phase I Detoxification ⟶ **Excreted in urine**

Phase II Detoxification ⟶ **Excreted in urine or in bile to gut**

Any of these pathways can be blocked by:

- **vitamin deficiency**
- **mineral deficiency**
- **amino acid deficiency**
- **fatty acid deficiency**
- **foreign chemicals**
- **newly formed metabolites**
- **enzymes poisoned by heavy metals**
- **excess body fat and inflammatory toxins**
- **mitochondrial toxins**
- **overload from everyday chemicals (total toxic load)**
- **poor genetics**

only using up vital detoxifying nutrients but also leading to fibromyalgia, allergies, asthma, skin rashes, chronic fatigue, and a host of autoimmune diseases, as they produce silent inflammation throughout the body.

The effect of toxins in any individual is determined in part by the genetics of that person's detoxifying systems (Phase I and II and other liver-detoxifying pathways). Although there are seven primary organs of elimination, most physicians would agree that the liver is the most important detoxifier. A properly functioning liver can clear 99 percent of toxins from the blood before they go on to harm the rest of the body. Although every cell in the body has the ability to perform Phase I and Phase II detoxification, it is the liver which is by far the most active in this process. Liver comes from an old English word which means "life." Your quality and length of life literally depends on your liver.

One of the most critical problems with obesity is the problem of non-alcoholic steatohepatitis, which now affects a large part of the population. The major feature is fat and inflammation in the liver. This condition is often silent and can progress to cirrhosis. In addition, it severely impairs detoxification. (Alkaline water, such as LIV Water, may have a dramatic healing effect on this fatty liver problem.) In a similar mode, chronic constipation can lead to increased resorption of toxins, further amplifying a person's toxic load. Remember, too, that obese individuals store and release more toxins because they generally have more fat.

ARE YOU TOXIC?

The chemical cocktail of stress, pesticides, industrial wastes, poor diet, heavy metals, chronic infections, and drugs greatly contribute to the silent inflammation in our bodies as we age. As the toxic load increases, so does inflammation and the incidence of most chronic disease.

Although scientists have been measuring the amount of industrial pollutants in the air, water, soil, and food for several decades, we have only just begun to measure the levels of toxins in tissues of the human body (known as toxic load or body burden). Recently, in the Human Toxome Project, seventy-five participants ranging in age from newborn to the elderly, all tested positive for 455 out of the 528 chemicals tested (including pesticides, heavy metals, and others).[9] Every citizen of an industrialized nation now carries over 700 synthetic chemicals in their body, and for most of them, the health effects are unknown.

Total-Body Toxic Load Test

Take the Total-Body Toxic Load Test to see how toxic you are. Answer the following questions "yes" or "no."

- Are you overweight? YES NO
- Are you constipated? YES NO
- Have you had hepatitis or other liver disease? YES NO
- Do you have allergies? YES NO
- Do you have your clothes dry cleaned? YES NO
- Do you live in a "tight" building without fresh air? YES NO
- Do you have one or more silver amalgams? YES NO
- Do you eat large fish more than once a week? YES NO
- Do you drink city water? YES NO
- Do you rarely sweat? YES NO
- Do you have chronic fatigue syndrome or fibromyalgia? YES NO
- Do you have concentration or memory problems? YES NO
- Do you chronically feel tired? YES NO
- Do you use commercial (non-organic) cleaners? YES NO
- Do you use regular deodorants? YES NO
- Do you take medications regularly? YES NO
- Do you use pesticides? YES NO

• Do you use air fresheners?	YES	NO
• Do you use cosmetics with coloring or fragrances?	YES	NO
• Do you use antiseptic soap?	YES	NO
• Do you have more than two alcoholic drinks a day?	YES	NO
• Do you smoke?	YES	NO
• Are you around a lot of second-hand smoke?	YES	NO
• Do you eat mostly non-organic food?	YES	NO
• Do you live in a large urban or industrial area?	YES	NO
• Do you wear synthetic materials like polyester?	YES	NO
• Do you use insecticides?	YES	NO
• Have you had a new car in the last five years?	YES	NO
• Do you have carpet at home or the office?	YES	NO
• Do you have a family history of Alzheimer's disease?	YES	NO
• Do you have a family history of any other neurological disease?	YES	NO
• Do you have a history of breast or prostate cancer?	YES	NO
• Do you have a history of bowel disease?	YES	NO
• Are you sensitive to any smells?	YES	NO
• Do you have any allergies to foods?	YES	NO
• Do you drink more than three cups of coffee per day?	YES	NO
• Do you drink out of plastic bottles?	YES	NO
• Do you have more than one electrical appliance in the bedroom?	YES	NO
• Do you microwave with plastic wrappings?	YES	NO
• Do you have chronic muscle or joint pain?	YES	NO
• Do you crave foods, especially refined carbohydrates?	YES	NO
• Do you have trouble sleeping?	YES	NO

• Do you have bad breath or body odor?	YES	NO
• Do you feel depressed or moody?	YES	NO
• Do you have strong-smelling urine?	YES	NO
• Do you often feel stressed and anxious?	YES	NO
• Do you eat fast food more than two times per week?	YES	NO
• Do you dye or bleach your hair?	YES	NO
• Do you use recreational drugs?	YES	NO
• Do you get more than 1–2 colds per year?	YES	NO

To determine your toxicity level, count your total "yes" answers. If your score is less than 10, you have minimal toxicity; 10–25 is moderate toxicity; and over 25 represents severe toxicity. There are several excellent laboratories that perform testing on individuals thought to have a toxic body burden. Although many of these tests are not well-known by allopathic physicians, they have been used for many decades to arrive at conclusive evidence of toxins afflicting individuals. (Our website, Inflamaging.com, contains more information on these tests.)

Toxins stored in the body can eventually overwhelm the liver and other body defenses. Since the liver is our primary defense against toxins, if it is overworked, an extra load is placed on our other organs of detoxification. Either balance is re-established or degeneration sets in (toxic stress cycle). The result of this toxic overload is silent inflammation, which is the underlying cause of most chronic disease and aging. These stealth-like toxins can lie dormant for many years, slowly accumulating until they reveal themselves through sudden or chronic illness. For example, Alzheimer's, which fifteen years ago only afflicted a half-million Americans, now afflicts 5 million. Partly to blame is the graying of America, but so too is the ever-increasing toxic load of chemicals known to cause widespread brain damage. The key is to make lifestyle changes to prevent this ill health from ever taking hold.

Signs of a Sluggish and/or Dysfunctional Liver

- Poor skin tone and sallow coloring
- Yellow-coated tongue or bitter taste in mouth
- Dark circles under eyes or yellow discoloration of eyes
- Liver spots (brown spots on skin)
- Acne rosacea (redness around nose and cheeks)
- Itchy skin
- Headaches
- Moodiness and irritability
- Excessive sweating
- Arthritis
- Flushed face or excessive facial blood vessels
- Red palms and soles (may be itchy and inflamed)
- Trouble digesting fats (chronic indigestion)[10]

Toxins Disrupt Weight Control

Although I have previously outlined the principal cause of obesity—insulin and inflammation—a secondary factor of great importance is the role that toxins play in weight control. Organochlorines, like DDT, first appeared on the market after World War Two and were used in agriculture and in the public health control of vectors of disease, such as mosquitoes. They were popular because they worked and they were cheap. However, many adverse effects have been associated with organochlorines, which are endocrine disruptors and enzyme inducers: they have been associated with some types of cancer (breast), with alterations in immune function, and with impairment of thyroid function.

In regard to weight loss, organochlorines come out of the fat tissues and can decrease thyroid function, resting metabolic rate, and skeletal muscle markers for oxidation of fatty acids. Could it be that the frequent plateaus often seen in dieting are due to these toxins poisoning our endocrine system? Researchers have reviewed more than sixty scientific studies showing a link between chemical toxins and obesity and found many ways that toxins interfere with our metabolism. Mark Hyman, M.D., in his book *Ultrametabolism*, cites a study in which an increase in toxins during weight loss in men inhibited mitochondrial function and reduced the subject's ability to burn calories, retarding further weight loss.[11] Toxins (such as heavy metals and chemicals) can also disrupt the hormonal signals (estrogens, testosterone, cortisol, insulin, growth hormone, thyroid, and leptin) that control your appetite and eating behavior.[12] Over time, your brain can become leptin resistant, so you are hungry all the time. Slow, steady weight loss with a detoxification protocol is ideal to avoid any adverse effects from organochlorines, PCBs, and other toxins.

HOW CAN YOU DETOXIFY?

1. Confirm You are Toxic

Review your history and the Total-Body Toxic Load Test. An examination and select laboratory tests will confirm your toxicity level. Develop a plan to detoxify.

2. Identify Toxins in Your Environment

Do a room-by-room evaluation of your home and office, paying special attention to the kitchen, bathroom, and bedroom. Don't use toxic cleaners, especially in the bedroom, as you will lie all night inhaling toxic chemicals and awaken with a fatigued detox system. Get rid of EMF appliances in the bedroom, particularly those close to your head. Select all future products with awareness and phase out your unhealthy products.

3. Clean Up Your Air

Use plants such as spider plants, ferns, and philodendrons to filter toxins from your air. Avoid air fresheners and other chemicals that will make your air toxic. Use an air purifier in the bedroom. More than 90 percent of particulates can be handled by a HEPA (high-efficiency particle absorption) filter. Regularly open the windows and allow some good cross-ventilation. Don't jog or exercise near highways. Clean and monitor your heating system. Air out your dry cleaning.

4. Clean Up Your Water

Either buy a total household water filter or install one on each faucet. Reverse osmosis filters lower the pH of water. Consider installing a LIV Water system (www.spaceaqua.com). Ask your water utility for a copy of their annual water quality report. For further options, contact the NSF Consumer Affairs Office at 877-867-3435.

5. Clean Up Your Diet

Follow the Paleolithic diet. Eat organic whenever possible and avoid all processed and fast foods. Go easy on coffee and alcohol, but drink

Powerful Detoxifying Foods

Cruciferous vegetables	Green tea	Fenugreek
Milk thistle	Wormwood	Flax seed
Radishes	Artichokes	Red clover
Hawthorn berry	Parsley	Ashwagandha
Cilantro	Yarrow	Chlorella
Kelp	Dandelion greens	Cape aloe
Citrus peels	Nettle	Beet
Oregano	Pomegranate	Ginger
Watercress	Horsetail	Slippery elm
Turmeric	Willowbark	Açaí berry

plenty of alkaline water and green tea. Choose foods that will help you detoxify. Remember to use nontoxic kitchen utensils—no aluminum pots.

6. Get Down to Your Ideal Weight

The greater your percent of body fat, the greater the amount of toxins that will be released and the more inflammation that will be generated. This inflammation causes more weight gain and a vicious cycle begins. You must break this cycle. Remember, the key is to reduce your glycemic load and insulin.

7. Sweat Out Toxins

Saunas are a great way to eliminate toxins by sweating. Far-infrared (FIR) saunas are safe and effective for this purpose. FIR saunas were used initially in Japan and entered the U.S. market in the early 1980s. They induce three times the sweat volume as a traditional sauna at a far more tolerable temperature. The sauna is ideal for detoxifying and has many other beneficial properties.

8. Exercise Regularly

Besides being important for weight maintenance, exercise is another way to sweat out toxins. Yoga and massage can also help move toxins out of your system. Bouncing on a trampoline (rebounding) is especially good at stimulating lymphatic drainage.

9. Enhance Digestion with Enzymes and Probiotics

If you suffer from chronic digestive problems, such as acid reflux, irritable bowel, or constipation, I suggest adding digestive enzymes and probiotics (friendly bacteria that can help re-balance your intestinal ecology).

10. Detoxify Your Body

The average man uses a fragrant shampoo, conditioner, mousse, shaving cream, toothpaste, aftershave, deodorant, and skin lotions, all containing chemical fragrances, colors, cleaning agents, and petrocarbon additives. Clothes contain odors from detergents and fabric softeners, not to mention formaldehyde and other chemicals to make them color-fast and wrinkle resistant. Chemicals in dry cleaning fluid, moth balls, and shoe polish can harm the brain.

11. Detoxify Your Mind

Worldview is essential to well-being, as I will show you in Chapter 8. A toxic mind filled with grief, fear, sadness, anger, and jealousy can hurt you just as quickly as DDT. Relaxation, laughter, joy, and gratitude are great detoxifiers.

12. Add Nutraceuticals

Take a good multivitamin/multimineral as well as anti-inflammatory nutraceuticals to help you detoxify.

13. Enjoy a Daily "Detox Cocktail"

There are several supplements that help detoxify the body, such as lipoic acid and milk thistle. Taking these types of nutraceuticals provide a cocktail that helps both Phase I and II detoxification.

14. Take Fiber Each Day

A good fiber intake (35 grams daily) is important to help cleanse the bowel. Both soluble and insoluble fiber help detoxify you. Eating a Paleolithic diet will ensure a healthy intestinal transit time (bowel regularity).

15. Consider Removing Your Dental Amalgams

Before removing your silver amalgams, contact Doctors Data and have a provocative heavy metal test done to check if you are mercury toxic. Mercury is especially toxic to the brain and heart. Oral chelators are powerful and inexpensive. Non-prescription alternatives are also excellent for the removal of mercury, lead, cadmium, aluminum, tin, arsenic, antimony, and more.

16. Avoid All Drugs

Try to avoid not only recreational drugs but all pharmaceutical drugs and the many over-the-counter drugs.

17. Take Omega-3 Fish Oils Daily

Omega-3 fish oils are one of the most important supplements you can take. Always be sure to use pharmaceutical-grade fish oil to minimize mercury and other pollutants. It is essential for controlling silent inflammation.

18. Consider Colon Hydrotherapy

Colon hydrotherapy (using water to flush the colon) was used in ancient Egypt and in most cultures. There is no odor and no risk if a licensed colon therapist is selected. The International Association for Colon Therapy (IACT) in San Antonio, Texas, is the worldwide licensing body for colon therapists; contact them at 210-366-2888.

19. Relaxation, Meditation, and Sleep

Healthy sleep patterns, making time to relax, and developing a meditation ritual will help detoxify the mind and energize your spirit.

20. Don't Forget to Breathe

Diaphragmatic breathing can be an exercise for relaxation and meditation in itself. The act of deep breathing will also stimulate lymphatic flow and help eliminate toxins.

21. Ground Yourself

In his new book, *Earthing,* my colleague Dr. Stephen Sinatra explains how simply using a "silver" impregnated bedsheet will help you sleep better, lower your cortisol, help thin your blood, and offer a host of other health benefits.

SUMMARY

Ninety-eight percent of the atoms in your body are replaced each year. We have a remarkable ability to rejuvenate ourselves when properly detoxified and nourished. In order to achieve optimal results, we need to pay attention to all our channels of elimination. These include the liver, gastrointestinal tract, lungs, kidneys, the skin, the blood, and the lymph.

CHAPTER 4

Exercise

"When you gain control of your body,
you will gain control of your life."
—BILL PHILLIPS, *BODY FOR LIFE*

FITNESS, IN ITS SIMPLEST USE, MEANS CAPABILITY. Applied then to the human body, physical fitness refers to the capability of the human body. But capability to do what? Generally, it is capability to maintain a state of health and wellbeing. Specifically, it refers to aptness for certain tasks. In terms of a Wellman, physical fitness means the capability to do anything you set your mind to:

• Perform day to day tasks with ease

• Have the capacity to handle any stress

• Have a vigorous sex life

• Play with children and grand children

• Run a marathon or a triathlon

• Have positive self esteem

• Sleep soundly

• Live without chronic disease

Physical fitness means having capability with utmost integrity; it means you have total control of your body. Originally, physical fitness was simply defined as the capacity to carry out the day's activities without undue fatigue. However, this definition has been insufficient since the industrial revolution because automation and computers have drastically reduced the amount of energy expended on a daily basis while leisure time has increased remarkably. Now, physical fitness is more accurately considered a measure of the body's capability to function efficiently and effectively in work *and* leisure. When you are physically fit, your body is an efficient tool that can be and is used to facilitate completion of your goals—and not just in terms of getting things done, but getting things done well.

Physical fitness does not just happen on blind accord, however. It is acquired through regimented training, aka exercise. It is important to note that exercise is different from physical activities performed on a day to day basis, often referred to as "Activities of Daily Living" (ADLs). ADLs include things such as climbing the stairs to the office, raking leaves in the yard, and other activities that require physical energy, but are not described by dedicated time and energy for training and conditioning the body. Both ADLs and exercise contribute to physical fitness. However, ADLs *maintain* while exercise *enhances*. In order to become and stay physically fit, it is important to not only have a lifestyle that is physically active (lots of ADLs), but also includes exercise as one of its key components.

HEALTH BENEFITS

Depending on how you define physical fitness, the corresponding benefits are innumerable. Because of this, The President's Council on Physical Fitness and Sports does not even provide one singular view of fitness but rather classifies as shown in the table on the following page.

Just as there is no one type of fitness, neither is there one singular benefit. Rather, it results in an all encompassing improvement in health, vitality, and wellness. Even beyond those that you can immediately feel and see, there are underlying multiple physiologic and health benefits. Exercise isn't just medicine; it is the best medicine.

BENEFITS OF PHYSICAL FITNESS			
PHYSIOLOGICAL	HEALTH-RELATED	SKILL-RELATED	SPORTS
Metabolic (Insulin etc.)	Body Composition	Agility	Individual
Morphological	Cardiovascular Fitness	Balance	Double
Bone Integrity	Flexibility	Coordination	Team
Inflammation	Muscular Endurance	Power	Part Time
Endorphins	Muscle Strength	Speed	Full Time
Detoxification	Blood Pressure	Reaction Time	Life Time
Endothelial	Muscle Mass	Core Strength	Professional

Evidence promoting exercise has been mounting for years. The best part is that there is no age limit for reaping the benefits. A study that followed Harvard Alumni over a fifteen-year period showed that sedentary men of any age who adopted a healthfully active lifestyle could reduce their total risk of mortality by 51%[2]. The impact of regular exercise was also found equal to if not greater than smoking cessation.

Regardless of what type of physical fitness being pursued, the corresponding exercise it takes to get it will have, as recognized by the Mayo Clinic, unyielding rewards including improved mood, reduced risk of chronic disease, weight management, increased energy, better sleep, improved sex life, and the list goes on. . . .

Detoxification

As elucidated in Chapter 3, Toxin Reduction, our bodies are exposed to a high volume of harmful chemicals and toxins on a constant basis. By speeding up physiological processes, exercise increases the rate of both Phase I and Phase II detoxification. As body temperature rises, perspiration begins. Sweating is one of the most convenient, fastest ways to begin the cleansing process. Exercise stimulates the body to perform optimally. Toxins actually impair working muscles from working at maximum capacity by interfering with the chemical process of energy production. Because optimal function and impaired capacity are not congruent, the liver is stimulated to drive out toxins from the body. Exercise increases metabolism, which promotes toxin elimination through the intestines, kidneys, and lungs. It also increases blood flow which facilitates the entire process. If your toxicity score from page 77 was a ten or more, exercise in your daily routine is imperative.

Sarcopenia

Sarcopenia is the loss of skeletal muscle mass associated with age[4]. The underlying mechanisms include a decline in muscle fiber number and area, motor unit size and recruitment, innervations, capillarization, protein synthesis, and growth factor alterations[5]. Limits in muscle function can be as high as 25 percent by the age of 65 and 40 percent in a lifetime. Nevertheless, the primary cause of sarcopenia has been identified as a lack of stimulus secondary to a sedentary lifestyle[6]—not age itself. In multiple studies, individuals who've adopted and maintained a regular exercise regimen starting in their younger years had a lesser or negligible rate of sarcopenic muscle atrophy when compared to their non-active counterparts. However, this does not mean that sarcopenia cannot be reversed. Instigation of an appropriate strength training routine at any age can result in increased muscle mass and strength. Ultimately, regular exercise means a lifetime of physical activity, mobility, functionality, and independence.

Body Composition

Currently, over 70% of the American population is overweight and the rate of obesity is climbing at an alarming rate. Being overweight is associated with symptoms such as depressed mood, low energy, poor sleep, low sex drive, and constant hunger all the way to chronic diseases including diabetes, cardiovascular disease, and metabolic syndrome.

Exercise, done properly and frequently, causes an increased level of stress on skeletal muscle. This is a eustress, a good stress, as

The Ideal Body

An ideal body is an ideal composition while being physically fit and healthy. Ideal body composition depends on age and sex and can be correlated to health/fitness rankings.

BODY FAT STANDARDS FOR MEN				
AGE	VERY LEAN	HEALTHY RANGE	OVERWEIGHT	OBESE
20–40 yrs	Under 8%	8–19%	19–25%	Over 25%
41–60 yrs	Under 11%	11–22%	22–27%	Over 27%
61–79 yrs	Under 13%	13–25%	25–30%	Over 30%

Source: Gallagher et al. *Am J Clin Nut* 2000; 72:694–701

There are many ways to measure the physical dimensions of the human body: height, weight, circumference measurements, etc. However, these measurements are only applicable for defining health status if they are interrelated. For example, the most common way for epidemiologists to assess the health status of a population is to assess body mass index, or BMI. BMI is the ratio of weight to height squared[7]. It is used to classify people as being underweight, normal weight, or overweight. BMI is a good indicator for health status of a population, but it is not accurate for assessing individual health status because it yields an estimated value. The difference between muscle weight, fat weight, and bone weight are not accounted for. Therefore, for individuals, the best way to measure body fat is to do so directly, with technology such as dual energy x-ray absorptiometry (DXA)[8].

However, no one has a DXA at home so how can body fat percentages be monitored on a regular basis? The most accurate home measurement for body fat involves a few simple circumference measurements and a calculator:

Estimating Percentage Body Fat for Men

Step One: Measure.

- Take circumference measurements at the waist.
  Note: this is your true waist, measured in inches, taken horizontally at the level of the navel. This may not be the region of minimal width.

- Measure your current weight, in pounds.

Step Two: Calculate.

1. (Total Body Weight x 1.082) + 94.42 = Factor 1

2. Waist x 4.15 = Factor 2

3. Factor 1 − Factor 2 = Lean Body Mass

4. Total Body Weight − Lean Body Mass = Body Fat Weight

5. $$\frac{(\text{Body Fat Weight} \times 100)}{\text{Total Body Weight}} = \text{BODY FAT Percentage}$$

As a general rule, all Wellmen, regardless of age should have no greater than 20% body fat for optimal health. Body fat percentages can further be used to calculate guidelines for ideal body weight, a measure can easily be monitored at home.

Estimating Ideal Weight for Men

Set a goal for optimal body fat percentage. Expressing that in a decimal (i.e. 15% would be 0.15) and using Lean Body Mass from your calculation of Estimated Body Fat Percentage, you can calculate your ideal weight using the following formula:

$$\frac{\text{Lean Body Weight}}{1 - (\text{Ideal Body Fat Percentage})} = \text{Ideal Weight}$$

Adapted from: Wolinsky I, Driskell J. *Sports Nutrition: Energy Metabolism & Exercise.* Boca Raton: CRC Press; 1998.

opposed to a bad stress, which is distress. The stress is positive because the body responds to the microscopic damage by remodeling, which results in stronger muscle fibers[5]. These stronger fibers are characterized by an increase in size, density, and volume. Muscle takes a lot of energy to maintain. Thus, exercise has the unique ability to increase energy expenditure during the exercise itself and, by requiring stronger muscles, also increase energy expenditure while at rest. This means that the body is using more energy all the time. Because the quickest and easiest source of energy is stored body fat, the end result is weight loss. More importantly, by increasing muscle mass and reducing fat mass, exercise can optimize body composition. Optimal body composition is one of the most profound characteristics of a Wellman.

Psychological

The mainstream benefits of exercise are primarily physical. However, the Integral Health Approach takes into account the mind-body relationship and the summation of consciousness. Therefore, the psychological benefits of exercise are as important as the physiological benefits especially considering an outcome of wellness. Among those recognized by the Association for Applied Sport Psychology, psychological benefits include:

- Improved mood

- Reduced stress as well as an improved ability to cope with stress

- Improved self-esteem

- Pride in physical accomplishments

- Increased satisfaction with oneself

- Improved body image

- Increased feelings of energy

- Improved confidence in physical abilities

- Decreased symptoms associated with depression

In short, exercise creates psychological capability. Not only that, but it has been associated with improvements in anxiety and depressive disorders[11]. Furthermore, exercise is a form of meditation. The increased level of concentration and utilization of biofeedback induce an increased state of consciousness. Speaking to the mind body relationship, regular exercisers have demonstrated improved regulation of their autonomic nervous systems, allowing them to respond more appropriately to emotional and stressful situations.

Physiological

The physiological benefits are not related to performance, per se, but are pronounced on the cellular level through biological systems. For example, regular exercise has been repeatedly shown to increase insulin sensitivity and improve glucose tolerance. Together, this ameliorates the onset of Type II Diabetes[4]. Furthermore, exercise increases free-fatty acid mobilization from adipose tissue resulting in weight loss and improved body composition[5]. Couple this with an increase in high-density lipoprotein and a decrease in triglycerides[12] and the end result is improved lipid and glucose metabolism. Improvement in other physiological parameters including heart rate, blood pressure, oral temperature, skin temperature, and resting metabolic rate[13] are also associated with regular exercise. Exercise has the ability to morph the structure and function of cells and tissues to enhance the function of organs, organ systems, and the human body as a whole.

Disease Prevention

Medical professionals once discouraged individuals with chronic disease from engaging in regular, strenuous activities. This was based largely on the premise that there was simply not enough solid research about certain conditions to ensure that the benefits outweighed the risks. Now, we are inundated with information and studies about heart disease, diabetes, metabolic syndrome, and osteoporosis. There is still much that we have to learn and have yet to understand. However, one thing is blatantly clear: Exercise is not just medicine, it is the best medicine. Physical inactivity is now considered a major risk factor for cardiovascular disease, diabetes, and osteoporosis.

Current recommendations of the joint committee sponsored by the American Heart Association and the American College of Sports Medicine guidelines on physical activity specify that all healthy adults ages 18–65 should be getting at least 30 minutes of moderate intensity activity five days of the week[14]. Guidelines for those 65 and older and 50–64 with chronic conditions or physical functional limitations that affect movement ability or physical fitness are similar, but take into account specific aerobic fitness and physical capacities[15]. Individuals with chronic conditions are still encouraged to exercise, but will have moderated intensity levels and may require the supervision of a physician. By conditioning the heart and lungs, exercise not only prevents cardiovascular disease, but it reverses it as well.

The cluster of metabolic abnormalities (hyperinsulinemia, abdominal obesity, elevated triglycerides, and high blood pressure) that constitute Metabolic Syndrome are strongly correlated with low cardiorespiratory fitness[16]. Men who engage in one to three hours of physical activity per week are 60 percent more likely to have Metabolic Syndrome than those who participate in a minimum of three hours per week[17]. Accordingly, the guidelines specified by the AHA and ACSM still leave an individual with a 60 percent residual risk for metabolic syndrome. Modern medicine has evolved to embrace the benefit of exercise, but only to the point of marginally reducing risk of disease. An integral approach, on the other hand, promotes more regular exercise *and* an active lifestyle to prevent *and* reduce chronic disease.

Exercise can also prevent and reduce the prevalence of osteopenia and osteoporosis, a degenerative disease of bone that affects more than 50% of individuals over the age of 50. This includes both men and women. By stressing bone tissue through muscle contraction and impact, exercise stimulates stimulates bone to grow[18]. Many well controlled studies have documented that regular exercise of virtually any type is an amicable treatment for bone loss in both men and women[19].

BENEFITS BY TRAINING TYPE

Exercise for physical fitness can be broadly broken into two types of training: aerobic and anaerobic. Aerobic refers to biological processes that require oxygen[5]. These types of exercise are generally low to moderate in intensity level for extended periods of time. Common exercises include running, biking, swimming, and walking. These activities are often regarded as endurance training. Anaerobic, on the other hand, refers to those processes that do not require oxygen. Generally of a higher intensity, this type of exercise is performed to increase strength, speed, and power. Common examples include resistance training or cardiovascular training with high intensity intervals, such as wind sprints or hill running.

The benefits of exercise can be further accounted for according to which types of exercise being performed (see table on the following page).

In order to get the maximum benefit, it is important to have an exercise routine that includes both aerobic and anaerobic exercise with a goal of at least general physical fitness and ideal body composition. My general recommendation for a forty-year old is that 40 percent of the work-out should be anaerobic training and 60 percent should be aerobic training; a fifty year old should split his workout into 50 percent anaerobic, 50 percent aerobic; and a 60-year-old should do 60 percent anaerobic, 40 percent aerobic.

A WELLMAN PROGRAM

Volume

Exercise programs should be progressive, meaning the level of physical performance and fitness increases with time and continued training. The human body is designed to work efficiently. This is why it responds by growing stronger and faster when difficult exercises are performed. In order to maximize training adaptations, it is important to have an appropriate training volume. Training volume consists of Frequency, Intensity, Time, and Type of exercise, often referred to as the FITT Principle[21]. Frequency refers to the number

COMPARISON OF AEROBIC VERSUS RESISTANCE EXERCISE

VARIABLE	AEROBIC EXERCISE	RESISTANCE EXERCISE
Body composition		
Bone mineral density	↑↑	↑↑
Percent body fat	↓↓	↓
Lean body mass		↑↑
Muscle strength	↑0	↑↑↑
Glucose metabolism		
Insulin response to glucose challenge	↓↓	↓↓
Basal insulin levels	↓	↓
Insulin sensitivity	↑↑	↑↑
Plasma lipids and lipoproteins		
HDL (high-density lipoprotein) cholesterol	↑↑0	↑0
LDL (low-density lipoprotein) cholesterol	↓0	↓0
Triglycerides	↓↓	↓0
Cardiovascular dynamics		
Resting heart rate	↓↓	0
Stroke volume, resting and maximal	↑↑	0
Cardiac output, test	0	0
Cardiac output, maximal	↑↑	0
SBP at rest	↓0	0
DBP at rest	↓0	0
VO_2max	↑↑↑	↑0
Submaximal and maximal endurance time	↑↑↑	↑↑
Submaximal exercise rate-pressure product	↓↓↓	↓↓
Basal metabolic rate	↑0	↑
Health-related quality of life	↑0	↑0

↑ = values increase; ↓ = values decrease; 0 = values unchanged
1 arrow = small effect; 3 arrows = large effect

Adapted with permission from Pollock and Vincent.[20]

of exercise bouts performed; intensity speaks to the degree of difficulty; time is the duration of exercise; and type refers to the mode of exercise, i.e. aerobic or anaerobic as specified by resistance training, running, etc. Attention to volume is especially important because it may be a two-edged sword.

The location of the endothelium between blood and vascular smooth muscle is a transducer of mechanical and chemical forces. The frictional force engendered on the vascular endothelium by the flowing viscous blood is termed *hemodynamic shear stress.* Sheer stress is a critical determinant of vessel caliber and plays a role in vascular remodeling. Moderate exercise has been shown to improve endothelial function through release of nitric oxide (a vasodilator, antioxidant, and anti-inflammatory) and to help treat atherosclerosis. On the other hand, too strenuous exercise stresses the body with activation of NF-kB and causes the accumulation of oxygen free radicals. Thus, regular moderate exercise may be beneficial for diseases that have chronic inflammation as the basis for their symptoms, whereas too strenuous exercise may worsen the symptoms[22].

An appropriate exercise regimen will have an ideal volume of physiological and mechanical stress that induces the desired adap-

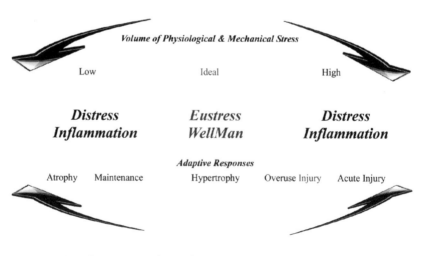

Exercise as a Stimulus and Correlating Adaptive Responses

tive responses. An inappropriate volume of exercise will result in distress, either from inflammation of chronic disease and atrophy or from biomechanical injury and hemodynamic sheer stress.

Application of the FITT Principle to training volume is a key component in creating a progressive exercise program. Any component can be adjusted at any given point to maintain an ideal level of eustress. This is especially important in the prevention and recovery from training plateaus and will allow you to maintain an effective, lifelong exercise regimen.

Creating a Program

Everyone has the same reason for not exercising: "I don't have time . . ." Modern life does, indeed, get busy with the business or work, family, friends, and general responsibility. However, the Integral Approach beckons us to re-examine our way of thinking about and regarding our own well being. In truth, the only people who have time to exercise are those that make the time. Once you start including exercise and increasing your capabilities, you will find that you have more time in other facets of your life simply because you are performing more efficiently.

Before You Begin . . .

The first phase of the Integral Health Program is to Measure. Because exercise is a stress on your body's physiological and biomechanical systems, before you begin an exercise regimen, it is important to have a thorough physical and health screening. By measuring and documenting your current health status, you will be able to ensure the safety and efficacy of your routine. Being aware of current medical conditions will allow you to modify your program to ensure it is safe and that no injuries/diseases are exacerbated. Measuring your current bodily parameters, such as body fat percentage, resting heart rate, and VO_2 will help you to properly set your goals and monitor progress.

With exercise, something is always better than nothing. However, the key to a successful program is to have a progressive program. This means incorporating regularity and routine. All Wellmen need to examine their schedules and prioritize time for exercise. Ultimately, the amount of time you dedicate to exercise depends on your goals and other life responsibilities. It is important to have a program that facilitates your goals and is maintainable on a day to day basis over the course of a lifetime.

Exercise

Exercise types are categorized into resistance, cardiovascular, flexibility, or balance training. Using the FITT Principle, any of these types can be performed as aerobic or anaerobic training. A well rounded program for physical fitness should include all of these types of training as well as a balance of aerobic and anaerobic training.

Resistance

Resistance training is a form of anaerobic exercise. It can be done with either an internal or an external form of resistance. An internal resistance would be your own body weight. Pilates, gymnastics, and yoga are forms of resistance training with an internal resistance. Training with an external resistance involves using free weights, dumbbells, and resistance machines. These are the training modalities most often seen in commercial gyms. Many experts believe that resistance training with free weights results in greater muscle growth as well as increased strength over what one can achieve with resistance machines. However, neurological adaptations are similar for all types of resistance training. Which type of resistance training is best for you is entirely dependent on your goals and preferences (see the table on the following page).

Cardiovascular

Cardiovascular training is aerobic training. Common modalities include running, biking, swimming, walking, etc. Again, which mode you choose is primarily dependent on your goals and your prefer-

In The Gym

As with any progressive program, there are many factors involved in creating a resistance training routine with free weights, machines, and dumbbells. First and foremost, the most important factor to consider is your goal. This information alone will depict the frequency, components, and duration of your work-outs. If you want maximal results out of your time and effort, be clear with yourself about your goals and objectives. If you only have one hour a day to exercise, it would not make sense to make a goal of completing an IronMan Triathlon. On the other hand, if you have a goal of general health and physical fitness, you won't need to a lot two-plus hours of training per day. Below is a sample of weight lifting variables manipulated by goal[23].

RESISTANCE TRAINING GOAL				
VARIABLE	STRENGTH	POWER	HYPERTROPHY	ENDURANCE
Sessions per muscle group per week	3–6	3–6	5–7	8–14
Sets per exercise	4–7	3–5	4–8	2–4
Repetitions per set	1–5	1–5	6–12	15–60
Rest between sets (minutes)	2–6	2–6	2–5	1–2
Load (% of one rep maximum)	80–90	70–90	60–80	40–60
Duration (seconds per set)	5–10	4–8	20–60	80–150
Speed per rep (% of maximum)	60–100	90–100	60–90	60–80

All these variables—number of exercises, sets, repetitions, rest, weight, duration, and speed—should be adjusted to accomplish your goals. Each variable should also be set so that it complements the other variables. For example, if you have a goal of hypertrophy and set your weight on a bench press machine to 150 lbs, but can only lift it once, your exercise is not conducive to your goal. A weight that would fatigue your muscles by repetition 8 or 9 would be ideal. For most Wellmen, a program reflecting a mixed goal of hypertrophy and endurance is appropriate.

ences. Cardiovascular training involves two primary sub-categories: steady state and interval training. Steady state training is performed at a moderate intensity for an extended period of time. The purpose of this type of training is to strengthen and condition the heart and lungs while improving endurance and stamina. Interval training, on the other hand, is a combination of aerobic and anaerobic exercise wherein one performs intermittent bouts of high intensity intervals followed by a moderate recovery period before the interval is repeated. The purpose of this type of exercise is to improve the rate of oxygen consumption and increase the limits of maximal performance. How much of which type of cardiovascular training you perform is dependent on your goals and physical health. However, a Wellman routine generally includes a combination of both steady state and interval training.

How Hard?

Intensity of cardiovascular exercise is typically gauged by heart rate. An Integral Health Assessment includes a VO2 test that measures your cardiopulmonary efficiency. This value can be interpreted to tell you exactly what your target heart rate ranges are for cardiovascular exercise. Target heart rate ranges can also be predicted, but keep in mind that predicted values are less accurate for people who are at extreme ends of the spectrum by either being very fit or de-conditioned. Using the formula below, you can calculate the low and high end of your Target Heart Rate Range[21,5]. For most men, the low training range is 50% while the high training range is 90%.

Target Heart Rate Range:

220 – Age – Resting Heart Rate = Heart Rate Reserve
(Heart Rate Reserve x Training Range %) + Resting Heart Rate
= Target Heart Rate

Steady state training best performed between 50–70% of maximum heart rate and interval training would include peaks of up to 90%.

Flexibility & Balance

Flexibility and balance are important components of physical fitness. Flexibility refers to the ability of a joint to move freely through a range of motion while balance is the ability to maintain proper equilibrium[21]. Training can improve physical performance, decrease risk of injury, improve posture, increase blood flow, and help maintain mobility and functionality. Training for flexibility involves two primary types of stretching: dynamic stretching and static stretching. Dynamic stretching uses speed of movement and momentum to move through a range of motion. Examples include drills that athletes perform before practice. Dynamic stretching is best included as a warm-up and should be part of every routine. Static stretching, on the other hand, is an active stretch wherein a muscle is elongated past its normal range of motion and then held for a brief period of time. Bouncing and fast, abrupt movements are discouraged. General recommendations are to stretch every major muscle group for 10 – 20 seconds. A static stretching session should be included as a part of a cool down period. Balance training is best accomplished by doing exercises that challenge the body's position. Yoga and plyometrics are common forms of balance training.

Components

A Wellman Program includes the actual exercise regimen *and* everything you do when you are not exercising. As much as 90 percent of results come outside of the gym. Exercise is the application of the stimulus. Results are the end product of physiological adaptation. Adaptation occurs when you are not exercising and it can only occur if you give your body the right conditions and the proper tools.

The conditions needed for physical fitness include those that characterize a generally healthful environment, such as minimal exposure to toxins and moderated social stress. By and far, the most important condition you can give your body, however, is rest. Muscles need time to rebuild and grow stronger. Exercise time and recovery time are positively correlated. The higher the exercise volume, the higher the amount of rest will need to be in order to allow adequate recovery and recuperation.

Nutrition, hydration, and supplements are the tools necessary for progressive adaptation and maintained physical fitness.

The best nutrition plan is a balanced diet of natural, nutritious food as recommended in the Paleolithic Prescription (see chapter two). This diet is more nutritious yet lower calorie than the modern diet. However, one major pitfall of new exercisers is that they think they need to eat more because they are expending more energy. This is not true. With over 70 percent of the population overweight, most people have more than enough energy stored as body fat. Exercise increases resting metabolic rate and trains the body to use fat for fuel. Ironically, even though a Paleolithic diet is fewer calories than the modern diet, you will have higher energy because your body is working more efficiently—just as it has been trained to do. Remember, a calorie is not just a calorie and quality is always more important than quantity.

High-quality dietary supplements, when used properly, can enhance an exercise routine. These types of supplements are called "ergogenic aids." An ergogenic aid is any substance that is endorsed as a performance enhancer. As outlined in chapter 7, Advanced Supplementation, all Wellmen should begin with a core program including multi-vitamins, Marine Plasma, antioxidants, fish oil, probiotics, vitamin D3, and enzymes. By contributing to a foundation of health and wellness on a cellular level, these nutrients could actually be considered ergogenic aids in themselves. Otherwise, the most common and proven ergogenic aids include creatine, amino acids, and caffeine but many others are available. However, many of the "Sports Nutrition" products available on the market today are simply glorified caffeine products. In addition, ergogenic aids are not standardized and many products, such as energy drinks, protein powders, shakes, and gels are highly processed and loaded with pro-inflammatory chemicals and sugars. Therefore, it is best to seek the advice of a credentialed nutritionist when considering addition of an ergogenic aid to your diet. This will ensure proper dosage, nutrient content, and timing for maximal results.

SUMMARY

A Wellman knows physical fitness yields innumerable health benefits. Regular exercise is how to get it. An active lifestyle is how to keep it.

- Physical fitness refers to capability to perform effectively and efficiently in all aspects of life. The benefits of being physically fit contribute to all dynamics of health and wellness.

- Physical fitness is accomplished through an active lifestyle and regular exercise. Exercise is a type of physical activity that requires planned, structured, repetitive body movement with specified intention toward a goal.

- Regular, moderate exercise, promotes health by stimulating maximal functionality of the body's biological systems. With exercise, something is always better than nothing.

- Intra-abdominal fat and insulin resistance are part of "metabolic syndrome" which causes increased heart disease. Intra-abdominal fat can decrease by as much as 35% with exercise.

- Recent research has shown that exercise is the "best medicine" and can delay and prevent most chronic disease by improving endothelial dysfunction.

- A Wellman exercise program includes both aerobic and anaerobic exercise and encompasses resistance, cardiovascular, flexibility, and balance training.

- Aspects of a Wellman program include the exercises themselves but also downtime. Maximal results come from properly planned, progressive programs coupled with adequate rest, proper nutrition, and a healthful environment.

CHAPTER 5

Graded Aesthetic Enhancement

Research indicates that the effects of chronic, low-grade invisible inflammation is at the basis of aging and age-related diseases such as cardiovascular disease, diabetes, cancer, Parkinson's, Alzheimer's, and autoimmune disease—and even wrinkled, sagging skin.
—NICHOLAS PERRICONE, M.D.,
THE PERRICONE WEIGHT LOSS DIET (2005)

WHILE MANY WOMEN SEEK SMOOTH, WRINKLE-FREE SKIN, men typically prefer a clean, fresh appearance that retains the ruggedness that adds character and masculinity to the male face. Therefore, the approach to aesthetic enhancement must be gender specific. Men may wish to eliminate the factors that make them look old, tired, or angry but preserve the features that define masculinity. Male-specific aesthetics may include use of Botox, fillers, and skin surface improvements with dermabrasion or laser resurfacing. Hair restoration and body contouring are additional aesthetic procedures frequently sought by men.

The skin is the largest organ of the body, comprising 15 percent of the total body weight. It consists of three distinct layers—the epidermis, the dermis, and the subcutaneous fat layer. The epidermis is the outermost layer of skin. It is a tenth of 1 millimeter thick (half of the thickness of a sheet of paper). The major purpose of the epidermis is to form the stratum corneum, a layer of dead cells that acts as a barrier between the body and the environment. Essentially, it helps prevent water loss and is resistant to chemical, physical, and bacterial insults.

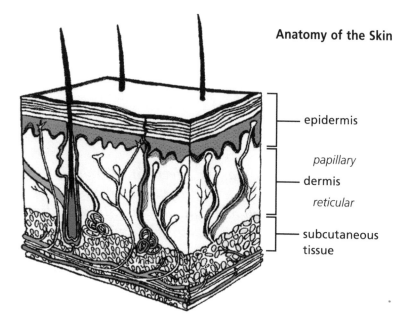

Anatomy of the Skin

— epidermis

papillary
— dermis
reticular

— subcutaneous tissue

Most of the epidermis is made up of cells called keratinocytes, which are formed in the basal (bottom) layer, one of four layers in the epidermis. Approximately half of these cells migrate up to the top layer, the stratum corneum, where they are known as corneocyte cells. The keratinocyte cells develop in a process called mitosis (cell reproduction), which occurs at the same rate that the corneocyte cells are lost. The usual time for this migration from the basal layer to exfoliation at the skin's surface is six weeks. If the skin is injured, the production of keratinocyte cells at the base level increases dramatically.

Melanocytes (melanin pigment cells) are also found in the basal layer of the epidermis and are connected to approximately 30–40 keratinocyte cells by finger-like projections. When the melanin pigment cells move through these projections into the keratinocyte cells, they form a protective cap over the nucleus (DNA) and protect it from ultraviolet (UV) light. Two other cell types are found in the epidermis. Langerhans cells originate in the bone marrow and are important for immune regulation. They play a role in delayed skin hypersensitivity, as do Merkel's tactile cells, which are felt to play a role in skin sensation generally.

The dermis consists of two layers, the upper papillary dermis (which contains the blood supply) and the lower reticular dermis (which provides strength and elasticity). Unlike the epidermis, the dermis has few cells—its master cells are called fibroblasts—and is composed mainly of connective tissue, collagen fibers, and elastin fibers. In addition to producing collagen and elastin, the fibroblasts also control the turnover of connective tissue by producing enzymes that degrade collagen (collagenases), elastin (elastases), and glycosaminoglycans (glycosomal hydrolases) to make room for new versions of these substances, important because their presence is paramount in maintaining youthful skin.

The innermost layer of the skin contains a single layer of fat that helps protect the internal organs. Blood vessels, nerves, and lymph vessels can be found here.

WHY SKIN AGES

As we age, a number of changes take place in the skin. Beginning at birth with the transition from a water to an air environment, and continuing with changes in hormonal levels, diet, and antioxidant levels, environmental toxins, illness, photo-aging (sun damage), trauma, and other lifestyle factors all play a role in aging the skin. And all this aging (blemishes, pigmentation, sagging skin, wrinkles, etc.) can be slowed and often reversed.

When we look at children, we notice that their skin is firm, smooth, and supple. This is because the skin is well-hydrated, well-oxygenated, and well-nourished. All the skin cells function properly and epidermal turnover occurs every two to four weeks (as compared to nine to twelve weeks in older men). This is partly due to blood flow and partly due to the higher concentrations of glycosaminoglycans (GAGs) in the basement membranes of the epidermis and dermis. These complex sugar-protein molecules can bind up to 1,000 times their weight in water and thereby keep the skin well-hydrated. In addition to their water-binding characteristics, they also provide a pathway for the diffusion of nutrients throughout the body.

Skin aging is mostly the result of inflammation and decreased blood flow, as, in fact, are most chronic diseases. Inflammation and decreased blood flow are primarily the result of poor diet and hormone imbalance. So, in addition to good skin care, a comprehensive skin program must focus on improving these essential elements. Although we cannot stop the progression of years, we can stop skin from wrinkling, sagging, and dulling.

The signs of aging, including wrinkling, crepey skin, sagging jaw line and jowls, drooping eyelids, and under-eye bags and puffiness, are all the result of silent inflammation. Our pro-inflammatory American "Krispy Kreme" diet, exposure to sunlight, smoking, environmental pollutants, and a host of other factors assault our cells and cause them to generate a cascade of inflammatory chemicals. This silent inflammation goes on day after day, year after year, not only causing us to feel ill (as it produces a host of chronic diseases) but also to look ill with aging skin and loss of hair.

Nicholas Perricone, M.D., author of *The Perricone Prescription*, was one of the first dermatologists to recognize the important link between inflammation and aging: "When I looked at a biopsy of skin that showed clinical signs of aging, inflammation was present. Yet skin that showed no clinical signs of aging showed no inflammation. This discovery so intrigued me that I began to search for ways to put my emerging theory to the test."[1]

Dr. Perricone's theory regarding inflammation and skin aging was built on the work of two other researchers, Denham Harman, M.D., Ph.D., and Imre Zs.-Nagy, M.D., author of *The Membrane Hypothesis of Aging*. In the 1950s, Dr. Harman identified free radicals as atoms or molecules that are missing one of their two electrons, thus compelling the free radical molecules to complete their structure. When a molecule or atom is missing one of its electrons, it is unstable and will try to take another electron from any other molecule in its immediate environment. In turn, the new free radical attacks a molecule next to it, and so on. Dr. Harman postulated that it was the damage to these molecules that caused aging. Free radicals are mostly derived from oxygen, which tends to lose an electron and become unstable. These solo molecules are called reactive oxygen species (ROS). The conversion of food to energy in our bodies is accomplished in tiny structures within our cells called mitochondria. The problem is that about 5 percent of the energy produced turns into ROS. In addition, free radicals are created throughout the body whenever there is trauma, exercise, infection, inflammation, or when the body is exposed to pollution.

Most scientists formerly believed that the cytosol (core of the cell) was the site of the majority of free radical damage. Dr. Nagy contended that free radicals were doing the heaviest damage on the outside of the cell in the membrane (the "membrane hypothesis of aging"). The cell membrane must remain "fluid" to function well, but as we age, membranes stiffen and lose fluidity. When this happens, nutrients can't get in and waste can't get out. The waste builds up and causes our enzymes to slow down until we are even unable to replicate our genes (DNA and RNA). Dr. Nagy realized that we had to protect the cell membrane if we wanted to prevent cell damage and aging from free radicals.

Antioxidants are the cells' free radical defense system. The cell membrane is composed of two layers of phospholipids. In order for the antioxidant to penetrate this fatty shield, it must be fat soluble. The cell membrane itself is also a source of inflammatory chemicals that can wreak havoc if they get inside the cell. When free radicals are generated from UV radiation, such as during a walk in the sun, those free radicals live for just a nanosecond and, as a result, they do very little direct damage. But these short-lived free radicals trigger the phospholipids in the cell membrane to break down into inflammatory chemicals. These are the chemicals (toxic oxidized fats) that can then leak into the cell and cause damage.

The interior of the cell is filled with a gelatinous material that houses the nucleus, DNA, and protein transcription factors. These proteins are tiny molecular messengers that can move to the nucleus to stimulate the replication of important proteins for cell functions. Two such factors are nuclear factor kappa B (NF-κB) and activator protein 1 (AP-1). These factors are not active unless the acid-base balance of the cell changes and free radicals are about to overwhelm the cell's defenses, a state called oxidative stress. NF-κB migrates to the nucleus and attaches to DNA, resulting in the production of pro-inflammatory cytokines. AP-1 migrates to the nucleus, where it causes the production of a variety of chemicals including collagenases, which digest collagen.

Our skin, chiefly composed of collagen, has no defense against these collagen-digesting enzymes. When collagen is digested, it results in the microscars that lead to wrinkles. By protecting the cell

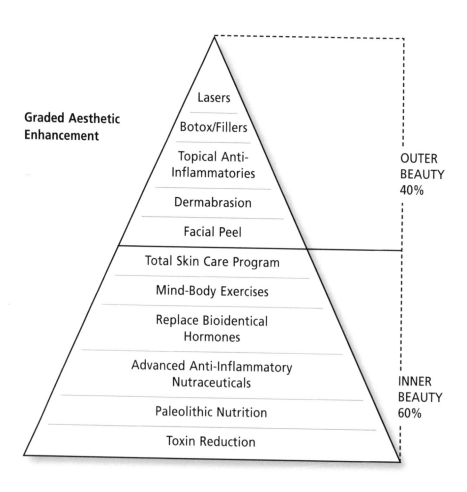

membranes and mitochondria, inflammation can be minimized, thus preventing accelerating aging. The Paleolithic diet, together with a host of anti-inflammatory nutraceuticals, a comprehensive detoxification plan, and select hormones, will have you not only feeling your best but also looking your best.

INNER BEAUTY

We believe that at least 60 percent of attractive and healthy skin and hair are created from the inside out.

Toxin Reduction

More than a third of toxins can be eliminated through the skin by bathing and sweating. Soaking in Dead Sea salts, diluted hydrogen peroxide, or Epsom salts will help clear toxins more rapidly than normal bathing. Alternating the water temperature between cold and hot will help activate the lymphatic system, which is designed to remove toxins from the body. Various types of bodywork, such as manual lymphatic drainage, also improve lymph flow. Body wraps (particularly those containing mixtures of aloe or seaweed) can enhance detoxification by stimulating lymphatic and blood circulation. Hyperbaric oxygen chambers use high-pressure oxygen to saturate tissues and help detoxification. Saunas, steam rooms, and far-infrared saunas are also helpful. Using a soft brush (vegetable fiber) during your bath or shower, or even ten minutes of dry skin brushing before a shower or bath, a couple of times a week can also be very effective for detoxification and skin health.

Paleolithic Nutrition

Once you accept that everyday lifestyle choices affect the way you age, you are on the way to restoring your youthful good looks. Food is much more than just a life-sustaining substance—it is our most powerful tool against inflammation and aging. The food choices we make daily directly influence the number of wrinkles and the amount of sagging skin in our faces. High-sugar (and thus high-insulin) diets cause the collagen in skin to crosslink, leading to the loss of skin elasticity and laying the foundation for wrinkles, sagging, and loss of skin tone.

Blood sugar reacts with minerals, such as iron and copper, creating free radicals that then attack the cell membranes, resulting in a cascade of pro-inflammatory chemicals, causing further damage and accelerating aging. To have youthful skin, we need a slow, steady release of insulin into our bloodstream. This is exactly what the Paleolithic diet accomplishes by excluding foods with a high glycemic index (above 50).[2]

Advanced Anti-Inflammatory Nutraceuticals

Alpha-lipoic acid is called the "universal antioxidant" because it is both fat- and water-soluble. It is 400 times stronger than vitamins E and C combined. Alpha-lipoic acid can inhibit NF-κB better than any other antioxidant, thus blocking the production of enzymes that damage collagen and preserving a smooth skin surface. It is also effective in blocking glycation, the harmful effects of sugar molecules on collagen. Alpha-lipoic acid will also selectively activate AP-1 that will only digest damaged but not healthy collagen.

OPC is the scientific name for an antioxidant complex derived from various plants, especially grape seeds and pine bark. OPC stands for oligomeric proanthocyanidins. OPCs in red wine are believed to help explain the so-called French paradox—that is, the French enjoy a relatively low rate of heart disease despite a diet high in saturated fats. OPCs are important in skin care because they protect collagen from free radicals, dampen inflammation, and help maintain the health and integrity of blood vessels.

Replace Bioidentical Hormones

As part of the many positive effects of hormone replacement therapy (HRT), there is improvement in skin and hair with growth hormone, thyroid hormone, and sex hormones. Recent research on thymosin beta-4, an extract from the thymus gland, has shown it to have powerful anti-inflammatory features and it also promotes wound healing.[3] HRT has a significant role in enhancing beauty from the inside out.

Mind-Body Exercise

Studies have shown that exercise can help the skin in much the same way that it benefits muscle and bone health.[4] The skin of athletes is thicker and has more collagen. All aspects of exercise, aerobic conditioning, flexibility, and strength training can promote skin health as well as an overall sense of well-being. Regular, moderate exercise is ideal to reduce the levels of the stress hormone cortisol and free radicals known to age the skin.

Someone once said that after the age of forty, we are all responsible for our face. For example, if you look in the mirror, you could very well have furrows across your brow (worry lines) or between your eyebrows (anger lines). Dealing with stress and maintaining a sense of equanimity is important for your skin health.

OUTER BEAUTY

Plastic surgery still remains the cornerstone for facial rejuvenation; however, recently a plethora of non-surgical treatments have become available that can provide excellent results with little or no down time. A good program pays attention to cleansing, exfoliating, hydrating, repairing, and toning the skin. In addition, you should always protect yourself from sun damage.

Protect Yourself from the Sun

There are three types of ultraviolet (UV) rays, UVA, UVB, and UVC. UVA rays are the second strongest burning rays of the sun (320–400 nanometer, long wavelength) and they penetrate through the skin's epidermis into the dermis. Through free radical action, they primarily damage the dermis. They also break down collagen and elastin, the connective tissues that keep skin firm and young looking. UVA rays, which penetrate deeper into the skin's layer than UVB rays, are associated with premature aging, skin cancer, and wrinkling of the skin. They maintain their intensity and wrinkle-causing effects throughout sunlight hours all year long.

UVB rays damage the epidermis. It is the UVB wavelength (290–320 nm, medium wavelength) that causes the tanning response and sunburn. They can cause premature cataracts and disrupt circulation and blood flow, which eventually leads to clumps of darkened cells (age spots) on the skin. UVB rays also increase the potential risk for multiple types of skin cancer. These rays, the third strongest type of rays, are most pronounced between 10 A.M. and 3 P.M. and are more intense during summer months, at higher altitudes, and in locations closer to the equator.

UVC rays are the worst, most dangerous type of rays (200–270 nm, short wavelength). We are protected from their damage by the ozone layer, without which we would not be able to exist on earth. However, 2–3 percent of the ozone layer has been depleted as a result of pollution. With time, it is hoped that this depletion can be reversed and that the layer can be regenerated to its full protective strength.

After years of research, it has been found that the best strategies for sun protection are the following:

- Avoid sun exposure during the most intense part of the day, from 10 A.M. to 4 P.M.

Types of Skin Cancers

Basal cell carcinoma—This is the most common type of skin cancer, affecting close to 95 percent of all those with skin cancer (more than 1 million people per year).

Squamous cell carcinoma—This is the second most common type of skin cancer and is more serious than basal cell carcinoma. Squamous cell carcinoma can be responsible for facial deformity and also has the ability to spread to the rest of the body.

Melanoma—This is the most serious type of skin cancer, causing more than 10,000 deaths a year in the United States. It manifests as a regular mole or nevi (birthmark) with tan or brownish spots and irregular borders. It has a hard texture and may cause itching and slight bleeding.

- Try to cover up. An act as simple as wearing a broad-brimmed hat can significantly reduce the sun's shining on parts of the body where skin cancer is most common (ears, lips, and nose). Wear long sleeves as well.

- When the above is inadequate (especially at a pool or at the beach), apply a broad-spectrum high or maximum sunblock to your face, each arm, and exposed areas of the shoulders and neck (when wearing an open-necked T-shirt). Apply the equivalent of 1 to 2 teaspoons to each leg and 2 teaspoons to the upper body when you expose more skin.

- Be aware of your skin. If you notice signs of short-term reddening or longer-term photo-aging (wrinkling or dryness), it is best to avoid further exposure to sunlight (even in the absence of such signs, it is a good idea to minimize your exposure).

- Visit a dermatologist on a regular basis.

Hair Restoration

Hair loss is a natural, daily occurrence: on average, 100 hairs are lost each day. When hair loss significantly exceeds growth, baldness occurs. In 95 percent of men, hair loss is an inherited trait caused by genetics. Until recently, it was believed hair loss in men was inherited only from the mother's father, but it is now understood that baldness genes are passed down from both sides of the family. People are born with a predetermined number of hair follicles that never changes.

While a child is in the womb, hair follicles are genetically coded. If the genes responsible for hair loss are present during this time, hair follicles are made sensitive to the hormone dihydrotestosterone (DHT). As men approach adulthood, the amount of DHT in the body increases, causing the follicles to cease producing hair. This process is known as androgenic alopecia (male pattern baldness). In androgenic alopecia, hair follicles that are producing healthy hairs begin to produce shorter, thinner, more brittle hairs. Eventually, these follicles produce only fine, almost invisible, short hairs or they stop completely (a process called miniaturization).

Hair Loss Drugs

Propecia—Propecia, manufactured by Merck, is the only prescription medication in the form of a pill approved by the U.S Food and Drug Administration (FDA) to treat male pattern hair loss. It works by blocking the conversion of testosterone to DHT, the hormone that attacks and destroys hair follicles. Propecia has proven to stop hair loss and, in some instances, re-grow hair in the crown. Based on clinical trials conducted by Merck during a 24-month period, 83 percent of men ages 18–41 with mild to moderate hair loss maintained their current hair count. The study also revealed 66 percent of men grew new hair in the crown.[5] Although these conclusions were reached based on a long-term study, Propecia can show measurable results in slowing hair loss within three months.

It is important to note that consistent daily use is necessary. If one discontinues taking the medication, all new hair generated as a result of taking the medication will be lost and hair loss will resume. Side effects of this drug are uncommon and do not affect most men. Women of childbearing age are not prescribed Propecia and instructed not to handle the pills due to the risk of birth defects in male children. Propecia is available only by obtaining a prescription from a licensed physician.

Rogaine—Introduced in 1988, Rogaine (Minoxidil) was the first drug approved by the FDA to treat hair loss. Rogaine is a liquid that must be applied to the balding or thinning area twice a day in order to be effective. Currently, Rogaine is available over-the-counter in 2 percent and 5 percent strengths. Rogaine products go to the root of the hair follicle and revitalize miniaturized hair follicles to re-grow new hair. With continued use of Rogaine, the growth phase of hair follicles becomes longer, and they produce longer, thicker hairs. Rogaine has been clinically proven to work and has a 64 percent success rate stopping hair loss and re-growing hair.[6] Like Propecia, it is important to remember that consistent daily use is necessary. If one discontinues using Rogaine, all new hair generated as a result of using the medication will be lost and hair loss will resume.

Low-Level Laser Therapy

While topical and prescription drugs help some individuals experiencing hair loss, they may not be acceptable for others. Now there's a new option available that is non-surgical and uses the latest low-light laser technology. According to *The National Hair Journal*, it all began in 1964 with Professor Andre Mester, of the University of Budapest, Hungary. While performing wound-healing experiments with laboratory mice, Dr. Mester discovered that low-level laser light exposure stimulated micro-circulation of blood supplies that regenerated tissues faster in wound healing. Dr. Mester noticed that body hair located in the region of the treated wound also grew thicker and longer than the surrounding hair. Low-level lasers are approved by the FDA for safety and for cosmetic enhancement, providing thicker and healthier hair.

Hair Transplants

The first step in advanced hair transplantation is the removal of a donor strip, a thin piece of tissue used to create the hair transplants to be implanted, from the back of the head. Technicians separate it into tiny grafts composed of 1–3 follicles. The next step is the creation of recipient sites (tiny openings in the scalp) in the area needing hair transplants. During a hair transplant procedure, the physician makes a specific number of these incisions based on each individual's particular hair loss pattern. Typically ranging between 1,000 and 3,000 sites, the size and spacing of the recipient sites are the foundation for a natural looking hair transplant procedure. Each graft is then meticulously placed at the right angle and depth into the recipient sites by a team of skilled transplant technicians.

After all of the hair transplants have been placed, the procedure is complete and the healing process begins. Because the graft recipient sites are small, they heal in a few days. The small clips that were used to close the skin, usually hidden by existing hair, remain in place typically 7–10 days. The final step is waiting for the hair transplants to grow. Virtually all transplanted hair follicles survive and eventually grow hair; however, the process takes time. Although some clients notice growth in four months, typically 8–12 months are necessary to witness optimum growth of their newly transplanted hair.

Except for a minimal amount of discomfort that accompanies the administration of a local anesthetic, hair transplantation is a well-tolerated procedure. In fact, most clients are awake throughout the hair transplant procedure and pass the time by watching a movie. Many people return to their daily routine within a few days. There are, however, recommended limitations on physical activity for the first two weeks. (My thanks to colleague Dr. Joseph Williams for his contribution on hair transplantation.)

Mesotherapy

Mesotherapy uses injections of pharmaceutical or natural ingredients into subcutaneous fat to induce lipolysis, the rupture and cell death of fat cells. In our male-specific form of abdominal lipo-dissolve, phosphatidyl choline (the active ingredient in all mesotherapy) is used to etch the abdominal musculature. Once a client has lost his subcutaneous and visceral fat, the abdominal musculature is further enhanced by dissolving the remaining fat in the tendinous insertion of the abdomen. This procedure produces so-called six-pack abs, adding the finishing touch to a fit male physique. Troublesome fat deposits elsewhere, such as under the chin and the common "handlebars" on the hips, can be easily dissolved as well.

PLASTIC SURGERY

Always consult with your physician prior to any procedure.

Facial Peels

It is recommended that extractions, masks, massages, and steam, in addition to the usual cleaning, exfoliation, hydrating, toning, and repair, be done by a trained professional. There are various facial peels to choose from, including alpha-hydroxy acids and beta-hydroxy acids, Jessner, or Obaji peels. Medical-strength chemical peels vary in intensity, depending on the percentage of active ingredients and different pH levels used. For example, you can achieve a medium peel of the skin after a recommended average of six peels (one per week). This will improve your skin's appearance and texture by removing superficial and medium wrinkles, diminishing acne marks, scars, and stretch marks, and improving depressed pits. This type of peel can also be done on the neck and chest area and on the hands. With a deeper peel, you can remove deeper facial lines that come with aging. After undergoing any of these procedures, it is highly advisable to use a high-protection facial sunblock.

Dermabrasion

Microdermabrasion is a technique that exfoliates the uppermost layers of the skin with precise control. The goal is to progressively treat and promote the cell renewal process, thereby stimulating the production of new cells. This will improve the skin's elasticity and texture, and result in fresher, healthier skin that looks better.

Topical Anti-Inflammatories

Alpha-lipoic acid (ALA): ALA is a universal antioxidant, both water- and fat-soluble, meaning that it is easily absorbed through the skin and works well as a free radical fighter, both in the cell plasma membranes and in the interior of the cell.

Vitamin C ester: The ester form of vitamin C is joined with palmitic acid, a fatty acid derived from palm oil, which helps increase absorption. The antioxidant power of vitamin C ester at the cell membrane provides key protection.

Dimethylaminoethanol (DMAE): As we age, loss of skin tone and sagging is due in part to the decline of neurotransmitters, such as acetylcholine, that stimulate muscle contraction. Studies have shown that DMAE lotion will tone your skin for 18–24 hours, causing an immediate reduction in lines and wrinkles.[7]

Olive oil: While olive oil is important as part of a healthy diet, since ancient times it has also been used as an emollient massaged on the skin. Historical records indicate that the Romans had beautiful skin, thanks at least in part to olive oil's powerful antioxidant and anti-inflammatory properties. Antioxidants known as polyphenols are contained in olive oil. They provide stability and protection for the skin and give it a smoother, more radiant appearance.

Polyenylphosphatidyl choline (PPC): PPC offers protection to the cell membrane. It can rapidly penetrate the skin and soften it while acting as a powerful anti-inflammatory. A natural moisturizer, PPC can reduce flaking and cracking in a matter of days.

Sunblock: Since most everyone is now aware of how damaging the sun's rays can be, it is vital to use a high-protection sunblock beginning at an early age. This is the key to preventing wrinkling, premature cataracts, and multiple skin cancers. The main ingredients to look for in such formulations are aloe vera, zinc oxide (micronized), phospholipids, titanium dioxide (micronized), grapeseed extract, wine leaf extract, green tea extract, sodium ascorbyl phosphate, vitamin E tocopherol, vitamin A palmitate, and mushroom extract. These substances will soften your skin and shelter it from critical moisture loss, while at the same time protecting you from aging and damaging UV rays.

Vitamin E: This fat-soluble nutrient is a powerful antioxidant and moisturizer. Vitamin E, made up of tocopherols and tocotrienols, is able to make hair shinier, reduce redness and flaking in dry skin, and prevent nails from cracking.

Topical vitamins (antioxidants): Vitamins A, C, and E, DMAE, coenzyme Q_{10}, and others are effective at promoting healthier skin.

Cell Therapy

Cell components from animals have been used to repair and rejuvenate damaged skin. We now use your own stem cells, harvested from your belly fat, and re-implant them in your face and other areas to rejuvenate the skin and other organs.

Fillers

Dermal fillers can be used before and between surgeries or alone. There is a large choice of fillers that are safe and very effective. Some last a few months, while others can last several years. They can also be used to enhance the lips. Fillers can be fat, collagen, or from materials such as calcium hydroxylapatite or stabilized hyaluronic acid. In this procedure, a filler is selected and placed in the area (for example, the naso-labial folds) by a licensed practitioner. This injection technique can cause some pain, swelling, or bruising at the injection site. The wrinkle filler Radiesse not only acts as a filler but can also stimulate your body to produce new collagen, giving a natural and more youthful look immediately. Other common fillers include Restylane, Perlane, and Juvederm.

Laser Treatments

There are laser treatments available for many different conditions, such as for removing acne, birthmarks, lesions, tattoos, wrinkles, or bulging leg veins or sun damage, and for resurfacing the face. Laser treatments should be performed by a trained plastic or dermatology surgeon who adheres to the standards set by the American National Standards Institute, the benchmark standards for safe laser use in the United States. Laser safety is based on the measurement of potential exposure risks identified with each laser's wavelength. Risk assessment is assigned by how the laser's wavelength interacts with the tissue, how it interacts when it strikes a reflective surface, whether it has the potential for flammability, and whether there is potential damage to eye or skin.

Botox

Botox is one of the few rejuvenating treatments that can benefit men of almost any age. It is also a preventive procedure against aging, because it will prevent the wrinkles that result from constantly frowning or raising the eyebrows. A Botox injection consists of a minuscule amount of the chemical secreted by botulism bacterium, but there is nothing alive in the injection. The small amount of botulinum A injected into select muscles weakens them. Its paralyzing effect does nothing to the muscle itself but rather works by blocking the nerves that supply the muscle. This effect will last up to six months, thus the procedure needs to be repeated. The only real side effect is a transient eyelid droop that occurs in less than 0.5 percent of patients. Some slight pain, swelling, and bruising may occur. It is a very safe procedure when done by qualified practitioners.

In the 1970s, Dr. Alan Scott, a pediatric ophthalmologist, pioneered the use of Botox to treat problems relating to vision. In 1992, a husband and wife ophthalmologist/dermatologist team first published results from their use of Botox for cosmetic purposes. From there, the field of Botox therapy advanced rapidly. In April 2002, Botox received FDA approval; there were over 2.4 million Botox injections in the United States that year. The only true contradiction is for people who have any neuromuscular disease or are on aminoglycoside antibiotics or who are pregnant.[8]

SUMMARY

- There are many non-surgical treatments that can enhance the skin of men while preserving the features that define masculinity.

- The major causes of aged wrinkled skin is silent inflammation, poor blood flow, and environmental factors.

- More than 60 percent of attractive healthy skin and hair is treated from the inside out.

- Paleolithic nutrition and sun protection are the two primary means of maintaining healthy skin.

- There are a number of options to prevent baldness. New advances in hair transplants give all men the chance to have a normal, natural, full head of hair.

- Comprehensive skin care programs for men help halt and even reverse aging of the skin.

- Recent advances in stem cell research holds promise that we can use our own stem cells to slow down aging of the skin and other organs.

- Protandim is an excellent product proven to reduce oxidative stress to the level of a 20-year-old (up to 1 million free radicals per second).

CHAPTER 6

Restore Bio-Identical Hormones

*More than two-thirds of all human deaths involve the
vascular (endothelial) system either directly or indirectly.
Signals (especially hormones) act on the endothelium
(input), are processed within the endothelium
(coupling) and enable the endothelium to
exert specific functions (output).*
—HELMUT AUGUSTIN, *ENDOTHELIAL BIOMEDICINE* (2007)

THE VASCULAR ENDOTHELIUM LINES THE INSIDE of all blood vessels.
The endothelium thereby acts as an interface between the blood and
the different organs. Collectively, the vascular endothelium forms an
enormously complex input-output system.

The inflammatory response is among the best characterized activation programs of the vascular endothelium. We have previously
discussed the role of high-glycemic foods and high insulin levels
that result in promoting widespread inflammatory consequences
throughout the body. In addition to the hormone insulin, other
hormones are involved in either promoting or reducing inflammation. For example, there are endothelial risk factors associated with
low testosterone. Testosterone levels begin decreasing in many
men during their late thirties. Low testosterone levels have been
shown to increase your chances of dying from heart disease and are
associated with all causes of death.[1] Older men with low levels of

circulating total testosterone had a 40 percent increased risk over the following twenty years compared to men with normal testosterone, independent of age, obesity, and lifestyle.

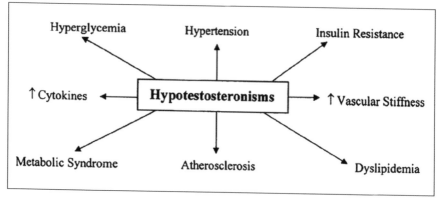

Hypotestosteronism

As we age, there is a decline in the levels of several of our hormones. Since the endocrine system is one of the key regulators of integrated biological function, altered hormone secretion and actions are important in the development of diabetes, metabolic syndrome, obesity, osteoporosis, depression, impaired cognition, erectile dysfunction, and loss of energy and strength. More than 40 million men are going through andropause (the hormonal changes associated with aging).

Hormone release is controlled by the hypothalamus in the brain. The hypothalamus, which is located at the base of the brain, communicates directly with the pituitary gland via special nerves and blood vessels. Pituitary hormones then work on target glands like the thyroid, adrenal, pancreas, and testicles. Different hormones are then released from these endocrine glands that have widespread effects throughout the entire body.

Hormones are the juice of life. Men are revitalized in as little as six to eight weeks after beginning hormonal replacement therapy. One of the problems I frequently see due to the excessive use of statins is low cholesterol levels. This is important when you realize that most hormones are derived from cholesterol. Our evidence-based wellness approach uses hormone modulation to help men regain and maintain healthy metabolic and endocrine function, adjusted for the patient's age—creating the best opportunity for a healthier and more vigorous life. Let's review the major hormones.

GROWTH HORMONE

Human growth hormone (hGH) consists of 190 amino acids and is secreted from the anterior pituitary. The hGH acts on the liver and

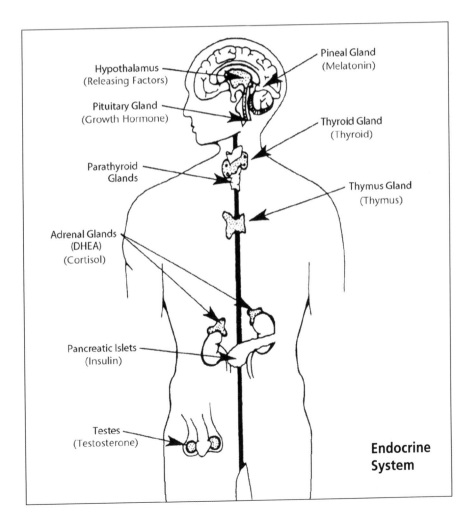

Hypothalamus (Releasing Factors)

Pineal Gland (Melatonin)

Pituitary Gland (Growth Hormone)

Thyroid Gland (Thyroid)

Parathyroid Glands

Thymus Gland (Thymus)

Adrenal Glands (DHEA) (Cortisol)

Pancreatic Islets (Insulin)

Testes (Testosterone)

Endocrine System

almost every other tissue in the body. It stimulates insulin growth factor (IgF-1) (Somatomedin C) production, and this in turn has numerous metabolic effects throughout the body. More than 20,000 clinical studies from around the world document the benefits of hGH therapy. GH declines with age in every animal species that has been evaluated. Growth hormone peaks in late puberty and begins to fall after age twenty; obese men produce less than lean men.

Daniel Rudman, M.D., studied twenty-one healthy men who had low IgF-1 levels (a good measure of growth hormone deficiency).[2] Twelve of these men received growth hormone injections over a six-month period, which produced remarkable results. Dr. Rudman showed that the signs of aging and those of growth hormone deficiency were nearly identical, and that by providing growth hormone to these men, it was possible to achieve improvement in these functions. Growth hormone has a wide range of potent effects on adipose tissue, bones, liver, muscle, the nervous system, and more. The broad spectrum of favorable effects helps us understand how different symptoms of growth hormone deficiency appear in adults.

GROWTH HORMONE CHANGES IN AGING			
FUNCTION	CHANGE WITH AGE	GROWTH HORMONE DEFICIENCY	GROWTH HORMONE TREATMENT
Adipose mass	Increases	Increases	Decreases
Bone density	Decreases	Decreases	Increases
Bone mass	Decreases	Decreases	Increases
Cardiac index	Decreases	Decreases	Increases
Glomerular filtration rate	Decreases	Decreases	Increases
Maximal breathing capacity	Decreases	Decreases	Increases
Muscle mass	Decreases	Decreases	Increases
Muscle strength	Decreases	Decreases	Increases
Renal blood flow	Decreases	Decreases	Increases

The majority of the effects of hGH work through the IgF-1 pathway. Until recently, hGH was considered a useful therapy only in children suffering from growth hormone deficiency, but in 1996, the U.S. Food and Drug Administration (FDA) approved hGH for use in adult patients.

hGH Therapy

We only prescribe hGH if our comprehensive evaluation reveals an adult growth hormone deficiency. Prescribing is based on multiple controlled studies in peer-reviewed journals in adherence with FDA regulations regarding the indicated use of growth hormone. An IgF-1 level under 350 ng/ml is generally considered evidence of a deficiency of growth hormone. We like to keep the IgF-1 between 250 and 325 ng/ml at our institute.

Since hGH is a protein, it cannot withstand a trip through the digestive tract because stomach acid and enzymes will break it down. Thus, hGH needs to be injected, generally subcutaneously every day in the morning. Growth hormone is made by the body mostly at night when we sleep, so we do not want to interfere with this production. We have not had much success using different sprays, creams, and other hGH look-alikes except for SecretropinRx. hGH releasing factor appears to hold promise in the future.

There are several factors that can help stimulate growth hormone naturally. First, dehydroepiandrosterone (DHEA) is a precursor and can help elevate growth hormone. Melatonin and vitamin D_3 at bedtime can help improve the quality of sleep and will therefore increase the levels of growth hormone. Better nutrition and resistance exercise can also help optimize growth hormone levels.

Growth hormone benefits may include:

• Fewer wrinkles

• Decreases body fat and increases lean mass

• Increases bone density

• Increases aerobic capacity

• Improves recovery from exercise

- Promotes faster wound healing
- Promotes better sleep
- Increases libido
- Improves cognition and memory
- Elevates mood and sense of well-being
- Stimulates immune function
- Improves cholesterol profile

Side effects of growth hormone therapy include mild fluid retention, joint stiffness/discomfort, may worsen insulin resistance, carpal tunnel syndrome (resolves with lower dose), and hypertension (uncommon). Absolute contraindications for use include anyone with a history of cancer (except skin cancer). Relative contraindications include diabetes mellitus.

MELATONIN

Melatonin is a hormone produced during the night from the pineal gland, located in the brain. It is made from the amino acid tryptophan, which is converted into serotonin and then melatonin.

Walter Pierpaoli, M.D., Ph.D., author of *The Melatonin Miracle*, has shown that the life span of mice can be extended by at least 25 percent when given melatonin. His research also showed that old mice can be rejuvenated by transplanting their pineal glands with those of young mice.[3] He believes that the pineal gland senses that we are too old to reproduce around age forty-five and begins to produce less melatonin. This signals all other body systems that the aging process has begun. Some scientists believe that a woman's larger pineal gland is the reason women tend to age more slowly and live longer than men.

Dr. Pierpaoli has found that by supplementing with melatonin, one can mimic a more youthful state. Melatonin will help the immune system by preserving the thymus, reducing levels of the stress hormone cortisol, and raising levels of the sex hormones. In addition, it is a potent antioxidant. More than half of the women with breast cancer have low levels of melatonin.[4] Melatonin appears to prolong survival rates with people who have breast, prostate, lung, and other solid tumors.[5]

Seasonal Affective Disorder (SAD) and Magnetic Storms

Psychiatrists have been baffled by the increases in suicides, depression, and anti-depressant drug prescriptions in September and continuing until March. Research by British psychiatrist Ronald Kay, of West Bank Clinic in Falkirk, Scotland, suggests that the explanation may lie in magnetic storms. He and other scientists investigating changes in the environment and their effects on human behavior are concentrating their studies on the pineal gland. Each year, the earth is wracked by dozens of geomagnetic storms (sudden changes in the earth's magnetic field caused by explosions of particles from the sun). Since these storms are most common around the end of September and the end of March, Dr. Kay was prompted to investigate and see if the correlation was coincidence or not. He gathered the medical records of patients admitted for depression to the Lothian Hospital, Scotland, between 1976 and 1986, and compared the number of admissions to records of geomagnetic storms. What he found was a striking correlation between individuals admitted for psychotic depression and increases in geomagnetic storm activity. In some years, the admissions during peak times of geomagnetic storms were up more than a third over average admissions.

Given this correlation, Dr. Kay is also concerned that electrical appliances could affect some individuals with depression, as 50-hertz electrical appliances have an effect similar to geomagnetic storms by causing small electromagnetic fields (EMFs) to occur within the home or office. Since any EMF can reduce melatonin levels in the body, I recommend removing as many electrical appliances from the bedroom as possible.

Melatonin controls the daily cycle of wakefulness. The pineal gland increases melatonin in the dark and diminishes levels in the morning with daylight. If this cycle is disturbed, it can lead to seasonal affective disorder (SAD). Shift work, jet lag, or any major change in sleep patterns can cause fluctuations in melatonin.

Melatonin Therapy

Melatonin supplementation appears to be very safe. I recommend using 3 mg (slow-release form) at bedtime. The slow-release form of melatonin helps you get to sleep and will also keep you asleep. Some people need much more than 3 mg, often up to 12–18 mg per day, an amount that should be used only under medical supervision. Calciferol (vitamin D_3), 4,000 IU and 600 mg magnesium, when added to melatonin relieves insomnia. Remember, insomnia increases the risk of dying in the next five years by 400 percent.[6] A few individuals will become excessively drowsy within an hour of taking melatonin, thus I recommend taking melatonin only before bedtime.

Melatonin's benefits may include:

- Protects against cancer

- May slow the aging process

- Improves symptoms of seasonal affective disorder (SAD)

- Preserves circadian rhythm; fights jet lag; helps sleep disorders

- Absorbs free radicals as a broad-spectrum antioxidant

Side effects may include drowsiness ("hangover" effect) and vivid dreams.

THYROID HORMONE

The thyroid gland sits like a small shield attached to the front of the lower neck. This gland puts out T_3 and T_4 thyroid hormones, which have many functions in the body. Adequate thyroid levels are essential to burn calories and provide energy for the body.

One of the most common (but often undiagnosed) causes of a variety of seemingly unrelated symptoms is an underactive thyroid (hypothyroidism). Broda Barnes, M.D., author of *Hypothyroidism: The Unsuspected Illness*, estimated that 40 percent of the U.S. adult population had this condition.[7] Some common symptoms of hypothyroidism include cold hands and feet, difficulty in losing weight, dry skin, low energy levels, memory disturbances, menstrual problems, mental confusion, overweight, poor concentration, and thin hair. Other symptoms include arteriosclerosis, depression, diabetes, hypertension, hypoglycemia, infertility, migraine headaches, and even acne. Correcting hypothyroidism can restore your body heat, emotional resilience, endurance, energy, mental vigor, and sexuality. It can protect you from cancer and heart disease and make your hair and skin healthy and strong.

Although many people exhibit symptoms of hypothyroidism, they usually don't receive treatment for this condition if their blood tests are normal. Their physicians often tell them that their symptoms are due to other causes or that their problem is "all in their head." Many are even referred to psychiatrists to treat their so-called psychosomatic problems. However, when they are later given thyroid replacement therapy, they improve dramatically. We refer the interested reader to Dr. Stephen Langer's book, *Solved: The Riddle of Illness* (4th edition; New York: McGraw-Hill, 2006).

Dr. Barnes realized that the usual blood tests to determine thyroid hormone levels performed by doctors are generally inaccurate. Consequently, he developed a simple test to confirm suspected low-thyroid function using an ordinary thermometer. He found that normal underarm or oral temperatures immediately upon awakening in the morning (while still in bed) are in the range of 97.6° to 98.6° Fahrenheit. He believed that a temperature below 97.6°F indicated hypothyroidism and that one above 98.6°F suggested hyperthyroidism (an overactive thyroid). For best results, repeat this test daily for three to four days. In my practice, I use the Thyroflex device, which can more accurately assess thyroid function than blood tests or temperature measurements.

Thyroid Hormone Therapy

Synthroid is the most commonly prescribed hormone for hypothyroidism, but it only contains T_4. The physiologically active form in the body is T_3, but with age and certain chronic disease states, many people have a problem converting T_4 to T_3. Thus, we have found it is very difficult to provide adequate thyroid supplementation with Synthroid without causing patients to develop a toxicity to thyroid hormone. Natural thyroid hormone, such as Armour, is a desiccated preparation of porcine thyroid glands and contains all thyroid hormone factors (T_2, T_3, and T_4). Unfortunately, many physicians have been bamboozled by the manufacturers of synthetic thyroid hormones into thinking that the natural thyroid products are an inferior, nonstandardized drug. Nothing could be further from the truth.

Most of our patients who switch from Synthroid to Armour report that they feel much better with the natural product. The dramatic improvements that many of them have achieved on natural thyroid therapy often appear miraculous. Often, they are able to lose weight for the first time in many years. Raising the body temperature by just 1°F (which can happen when taking thyroid hormones) equates to a fifty-pound weight loss in one year.

Occasionally, it may be necessary to take as much as 5 grains of thyroid daily (full replacement therapy) to obtain complete relief of symptoms. It is not really necessary to receive periodic blood tests, as it is more important to treat the patient than to treat the blood test, but performing the tests is wise from a medical/legal perspective. Using natural thyroid hormone is very safe. There is little risk of excessive thyroid dosage as long as:

- You feel well

- Your temperature remains below 98.2°F

- Your pulse is less than 75 beats a minute

- Your thyroid function tests remain normal (don't be fooled because most hypothyroid people feel best with TSH levels that are below normal). In fact, as a result of recent research, the upper limit of TSH of 5.5 MIU\L has been decreased to 2.0–2.5 MIU\L. People feel much better when their TSH is decreased to less than 2 by supplementing with a natural thyroid preparation like Armour rather than Synthroid.

Benefits of thyroid hormone therapy may include:

- Improves energy

- Increases body temperature

- Better skin, hair, and nails

- Better control of weight

- Fewer colds

- Increased libido

- Better mood and improved memory

- Better circulation

- Less pain and joint stiffness

Side effects may include a "wired" feeling (like having an extra cup of coffee), fast resting pulse, and insomnia.

DEHYDROEPIANDROSTERONE (DHEA)

DHEA is the most abundant steroid hormone found in the body. The source of most DHEA are the adrenal glands (located atop the kidneys), although small amounts are made in the gonads, skin, and brain. Many researchers believe high levels of DHEA in the body to be an excellent marker of general health. Studies indicate that DHEA has significant anti-aging, anti-cancer, and anti-obesity effects and that it enhances mental abilities. Again, like other hormones, DHEA levels fall with age, so by the age of seventy-five we only have about 10 percent of what we had at age twenty.

William Regelson, M.D., author of *The Superhormone Promise*, treated ten individuals with DHEA (1,600 mg per day) and showed after one month that a significant amount of their fat was replaced by

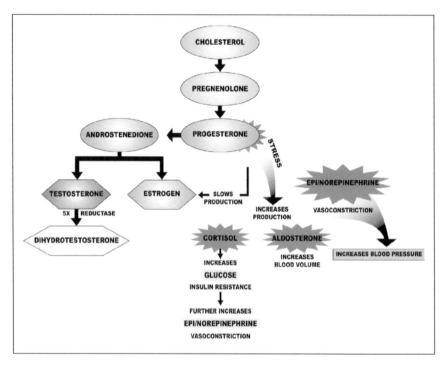

The Hormone Cycle

lean muscle. Their actual weight had not changed and there were no side effects. Another study showed that in a group of men aged 60–80, those with the highest levels of DHEA were leaner and more fit and had higher levels of testosterone. It is because of studies like this that DHEA has been nicknamed the "youth steroid." Low DHEA levels have been found in patients with heart disease and cancer.[8] DHEA is also a powerful immune booster and has potent anti-viral effects.

DHEA Therapy

I typically use doses of 50–75 mg of DHEA daily. Some clinicians will use 1,600–2,000 mg daily for those with serious immune disorders or human immunodeficiency virus (HIV). Smaller doses are effective if DHEA is taken sublingually or transdermally. DHEA cream appears to convert readily and to be 2.5 times more potent; this form (7-Keto) of DHEA apparently will also not convert to testosterone.

DHEA benefits may include:

- Improves mental and physical function

- Increases bone density

- Increases lean body mass

- Elevates mood

- Lowers cortisol (the "stress hormone") levels

- Provides protection against cancer

- Protects the brain from Alzheimer's disease

- Decreases heart disease (reduced plaque and sticky platelets)

- Increases insulin sensitivity

- Increases testosterone levels and sexual arousal

- Potent anti-viral effects

Side effects of **DHEA** may include increased facial hair and size of the liver (due to testosterone increase), and increased levels of the estrogen hormone estradiol (except 7-Keto DHEA, which does not convert to testosterone and thus to estradiol).

CORTISOL

Cortisol is one hormone that may increase as we age. We know that excess levels are associated with difficulty in losing weight and that high levels can also damage the brain. An extreme form of excess cortisol is Cushing's disease, which usually results from a tumor in the pituitary or adrenal gland. Far more common is Cushing's syndrome, which results from someone receiving too much cortisone (prednisone). What I would like to mention here is the other side of the spectrum—adrenal fatigue. Many traditional doctors do not give much credence to this disease. In my clinical experience, this is not uncommon and is more frequent in women.

Exposure to prolonged excessive stress (physical, mental, or emotional) can manifest with adrenal fatigue.[9] Some common symptoms include:

- Difficulty getting up in the morning
- Continuing fatigue not relieved by sleep
- Craving for salt or salty foods
- Lack of energy
- Increased effort to do everyday tasks
- Decreased sex drive
- Decreased ability to handle stress
- Increased time to recover from injury
- Light-headed when standing up quickly
- Mild depression
- Less enjoyment in life
- Memory is less accurate
- Symptoms worse if meals are skipped
- Thoughts are less focused

Adrenal fatigue can be treated, provided you are diagnosed. Besides lifestyle changes (only moderate exercise), you need to improve your diet and add adrenal extracts, nutritional supplements, and balance all your hormones, especially thyroid. Hydrocortisone (Cortef, 5 mg) used in the mid-morning and mid-afternoon can be very helpful in the right patient.

TESTOSTERONE

Testosterone is produced by the Leydig cells in the testes and peaks in the late teens. Men have about 700 million Leydig cells at birth, but this declines by 6 million per year after age twenty. The ancient Greeks were the first to describe the connection between the testes and male vigor. They noted these findings with male castration. The Roman physician Galen (129–200 A.D.) prescribed the consumption of animal testes in an attempt to restore vigor.

Andropause is the term for the changes that men go through as they age (the counterpart of menopause in women). Andropause (known in England as viropause) involves the progressive decline of testosterone levels with age, coupled with an increased production of sex hormone-binding globulin (SHBG). Testosterone binds to this protein, reducing its availability to tissues, and thus reducing its effect. Between the ages of forty and seventy, a typical American male loses about twenty pounds of muscle, 15 percent of his bone mass, and nearly two inches in height. After age forty, the testicles begin to shrink, so that many men become impotent in their later years. It is estimated that testosterone levels will drop to abnormally low levels in more than 50 percent of men after age forty, making testosterone deficiency a major unrecognized health problem.[10] In the last 800 men I have seen for age management, only about five percent had normal testosterone levels.

We do not believe that andropause is related only to a decline in testosterone, because higher testosterone levels by themselves do not always mean there is increased sexual prowess. Other hormones, such as DHEA, growth hormone, and thyroid hormone, are also very important in andropause. Sexual decline may also be related to a decrease in neurotransmitters in the brain. Certain medications can also aggravate brain neurotransmission and interfere with a man's potency.

Testosterone can not only be affected by medications but also by illness, obesity, stress, and lifestyle factors, such as excessive alcohol intake and smoking. Recent studies suggest that pesticides and preservatives in foods and the hormones used to fatten up cattle, pigs, and chickens can all act as "hormone disruptors."[11] It is also clear that as environmental pollution increases each decade, testosterone levels and sperm counts will continue to fall each year.

Determining Testosterone Levels

The following is a simple questionnaire for men to determine if their testosterone levels are adequate. Circle the correct response.

Do you have:

A decrease in sex drive?	Yes	No
A less strong erection?	Yes	No
A lack of energy?	Yes	No
A decrease in strength and/or endurance?	Yes	No
Lost height?	Yes	No
Decreased enjoyment of life?	Yes	No
Sadness and/or grumpiness?	Yes	No
A deterioration in your sports ability?	Yes	No
A tendency to fall asleep after dinner?	Yes	No
Decreased work performance?	Yes	No
Poor muscle tone?	Yes	No
Fat around your middle?	Yes	No
Seldom early morning erections?	Yes	No
Blood sugar problems?	Yes	No
Is your memory deteriorating?	Yes	No
Are you over thirty-five years old?	Yes	No

How did you score? If you answered "yes" to four or more questions, you are probably a candidate for hormone replacement.

There are more than 40 million men in the United States experiencing andropause, but the vast majority of them don't realize it. As the tremendous popularity of Viagra suggests, many of these men have symptoms of male sexual dysfunction, while others find themselves fighting more subtle battles against depression, diabetes, fatigue, insomnia, and obesity—all common symptoms of low testosterone that most doctors overlook and attribute to the natural process of aging or stress.

Testosterone Therapy

In 1889, British neurologist Charles-Édouard Brown-Séquard (1817–1894), thought to be an inspiration for Robert Louis Stevenson's character of Dr. Jekyll, gave himself crushed animal testicles and claimed that he became stronger, developed more stamina, and had a better memory. This is one of the earliest examples of a cell therapy treatment.

There are at least five common methods used to replace testosterone: creams or gels, lozenges by mouth, injections (SQ or IM), patches, and implantation of pellets. Our preference is to use injections. There are several forms of injectable testosterone approved for use in the U.S., both short-acting (aqueous testosterone, testosterone cyprionate, and testosterone proprionate) and long-acting (testosterone enanthate and deca durabolin) forms. Testosterone undecanoate is a new injectable testosterone that needs only four or five injections per year and will probably be available soon in the United States.

Another option is to use human chorionic gonadotropin (hCG). In men in their thirties and forties, the pituitary gland slows down or stops producing the stimulating luteinizing hormone (LH). The testicles are not receiving a signal from LH, so they don't produce testosterone. hCG given twice a week will increase testosterone production by the Leydig cells. And unlike with using exogenous testosterone, the testicles will not shrink. hCG should only be used if fertility is an issue.

Of note, testosterone replacement is key for diabetic men, as their testosterone levels are significantly lower. Testosterone treatment improves insulin resistance, glycemic control, visceral fat burning, and blood fats.[12] Testosterone improves the transport of glucose from the blood into the cell and enhances insulin sensitivity. Many people with diabetes lose weight with testosterone therapy and a low-glycemic diet. Many of these people are carbohydrate sensitive, with an exaggerated insulin response, so a drop in blood sugar triggers constant hunger and the need to eat more simple carbohydrates. Wheat and milk are the most frequent hypersensitivity foods and should be eliminated.

Laboratory Tests

When it comes to treating and eliminating the signs and symptoms of low testosterone, detecting the problem is a fundamental first step. In the healthy male, serum testosterone is present in three different forms: approximately 80 percent is strongly bound to SHBG; the other 20 percent is biologically active, some weakly bound to the protein albumen and some free testosterone.

- Total Testosterone: Deficiency is noted when the blood level is less than 350 ng/dL. We prefer the level to be at 1,000 ng/dL. Blood samples should be drawn in the morning because there may be significant daily variations in testosterone levels depending on stress, exercise, or other hormonal therapy. The goal is to restore levels to the high end of the normal range.

- Free Testosterone: Deficiency is usually present when the free testosterone is less than 50 pg/ml. We prefer the level to be at 200 pg/ml.

- Free Testosterone Index: This is the most accurate test: (Total testosterone [ng/dL] × 0.035) ÷ SHBG (nanomoles/L). The ratio should be 0.7–1.0. Andropausal symptoms are usually present when it falls below 50 percent.

- Follicle-Stimulating Hormone (FSH) and Luteinizing Hormone (LH): We find levels of these hormones above 5 MIU\L in more than 50 percent of men complaining of andropause. Normal values are 5 MIU\L or less.

- Estradiol: Estradiol is one of the active forms of estrogen in the body. A fifty-year-old male actually has more estrogen than a fifty-year-old female. The more obese the man is, the higher the estrogen level, because fat cells have increased activity of the aromatase enzyme, which converts testosterone to estrogen. This estrogen competes for cell receptor sites with testosterone. It is also important to monitor estradiol levels when supplementing with testosterone. If the patient notices a decrease in the effects of hormone replacement, it is often the result of increased estrogen levels.

- Dihydrotestosterone (DHT): We also monitor the conversion of testosterone to DHT, a more potent form of testosterone linked to prostate enlargement and thinning hair.
- Prostate-Specific Antigen (PSA) and Hematocrit (HCT): PSA and HCT levels should also be measured during testosterone therapy. The PSA level (an increase is linked to prostate problems such as enlargement or cancer) usually does not change. However, HCT (a measure of the volume of red blood cells) may increase; if it rises above 55 percent, you need to donate blood, decrease testosterone dose, or (rarely) stop the testosterone therapy.

Testosterone benefits may include:

- Improves blood sugar control
- Benefits cardiac health (improves high blood pressure, reduces cholesterol)
- Builds muscle mass and strength; decreases body fat
- Increases bone density
- Improves mood and sense of well-being
- Boosts energy levels
- Improves verbal and working memory and clarity of thought
- Improves erectile performance and quality of orgasms

Side effects of androgen therapy may include water retention, polycythemia (excessive red blood cell mass), hepatotoxicity (highest risk with oral preparations), sleep apnea, adverse lipid profile, gynecomastia (breast growth, nipple sensitivity), acne, hair loss, infertility due to a decrease in pituitary gonadotropin causing decreased spermatogenesis, and benign prostatic hypertrophy (BPH).

Contraindications to testosterone replacement include these absolute contraindications:

- The suspicion of, or already existing, prostate cancer or breast cancer (although some consider men who have had treatment for prostate cancer and no occurrence to be low risk)

- Obstructive uropathy

- Desire to reproduce (change to hCG)

- Hematocrit (HCT) above 55 percent

Relative contraindications include elevated HCT (52–55 percent); pre-existing cardiac, renal, or hepatic disease; sleep apnea or high risk for sleep apnea (chronic obstructive pulmonary disease in overweight persons or heavy smokers); and gynecomastia.

Men on testosterone therapy should at least take the herb saw palmetto (*Serenoa repens*) (160 mg) with pygeum twice daily, which blocks the conversion of testosterone to DHT. This helps prevent any complications involving the prostate (see table for other options).

A final note: erectile dysfunction (ED) and testosterone deficiency in aging men are separate clinical entities that often overlap. Androgen deficiency is quite common in men presenting with ED and correlates significantly with age, uncontrolled diabetes, hypercholesterolemia, and anemia. Androgen deficiency in the aging male (ADAM) includes ED, loss of libido, depression, lethargy, osteoporosis, and loss of muscle mass or strength. Guidelines have defined ADAM as a testosterone level of less than 200 ng/dL, plus one or more of the aforementioned symptoms.

ED is a disorder heavily weighted to the older population, with over 70 percent of cases associated with diseases such as diabetes, hypertension, atherosclerosis, renal failure, chronic alcoholism, and neurological disease. Since erectile function declines with age due to multiple causes—the most prominent of which is impaired penile nitric oxide (a vasodilator) release—ED may not be corrected by testosterone therapy alone unless the local vasodilatory defect is corrected first. But testosterone replacement may help enhance libido and contribute to improvement in sexual function in older men co-treated for ED.[13]

PREVENTING PROSTATE DISEASE		
AGENT	PRESUMED MECHANISM OF ACTION	FINDINGS
Finasteride	Inhibits 5-alpha reductase	25 percent reduction in total prostate cancer risk after seven years
Dutasteride	Inhibits 5-alpha reductase	Awaiting trial results
Selective estrogen-receptor modulators	Blocks estrogen-induced cell proliferation	48 percent reduction in prostate cancer risk seen in phase II trial
Selenium	Antioxidant; immuno-modulator; enhancement of apoptosis (programmed cell death)	Increasing amount of epidemiological and experimental evidence; phase III trial suggests 63 percent reduction in incidence (a secondary outcome)
Vitamin E	Antioxidant; decreases steroid hormone levels; anti-inflammatory; enhancement of apoptosis	Supported by observational data; one study has shown a 34 percent risk reduction as a secondary outcome
Soy phyto-estrogens	Blocks estrogen-induced cell proliferation	Increased soy consumption is associated with decreased early prostate cancer, but some studies disagree
Green tea	Enhancement of apoptosis	Lower incidence of prostate cancer in Asian countries may be linked to green tea consumption; minimal benefit noted in clinical studies in advanced prostate cancer
Lycopene	Antioxidant; enhancement of apoptosis	Some studies suggest it reduces risk, others find no benefit

Source: "Preventing Prostate Disease." *American Journal of Men's Health* 20 (November 2008).

SUMMARY

- The overall deterioration of the body that comes with growing old is not inevitable. We now realize that many aspects of it can be prevented or reversed by restoring our bio-identical hormones.

- Andropause (male menopause) is often not diagnosed, just as hypothyroidism and adrenal fatigue are often missed. Specific laboratory tests can help make a diagnosis.

- All the major hormones need to be restored. Bio-identical hormones are the first choice to help men regain their optimum health.

- When men are replacing testosterone and other hormones, it is essential that blood tests are done at least 2–3 times a year to optimize levels and prevent any side effects.

- Testosterone is essential to help men who are overweight or have diabetes or metabolic syndrome, as it can help normalize blood sugar levels.

- SecetropinRx will enhance ones own growth hormone and should be considered the first line of treatment for growth hormone deficiency.

- Erectile dysfunction is often the forerunner of heart disease. Infrequent early morning erections (in my opinion a better test than a treadmill) may be the first sign of ischemic heart disease.

- Most andropausal symptoms (over 70%) appear to be relieved primarily with testerone replacement. Growth hormone needs to be used selectively in fewer clients.

CHAPTER 7

Advanced
Supplementation

*Nutraceuticals can be broadly defined as
components of foods or dietary supplements that
have a medicinal or therapeutic effect. In general,
nutraceuticals are taken in amounts higher than
that which can be obtained from a regular diet.*

—ARTHUR ROBERTS, M.D.

SCIENTIFIC RESEARCH HAS REVEALED several theories of aging, but the
common link and final common pathway appears to be "silent
inflammation."[1] If inflammation is indeed the underlying cause of
most chronic disease and aging, then using advanced anti-inflammatory products is essential for optimizing health and extending life.

When we look at advanced supplementation, we need to look at
both our intracellular and extracellular tissues. There are 45 liters of
water in the body, shared among the cells (30 L), the tissues or inter-
stitial spaces (12 L), and the blood plasma (3 L). The water in the
cells plus their dissolved salts are the intracellular fluid, while the
tissue fluid and the plasma together constitute the extracellular fluid.

Most supplementation today usually only considers intracellular
nutrition. Recent research has shown that genes control physical
expression and only part of our health.[2] Cells also respond to their
environment, not just to genetic programming. The extracellular fluid
is the immediate environment surrounding every cell in our bodies.

Cells are not in direct contact with each other, and all intercellular information (nervous stimuli, metabolic, immunologic, and vascular processes, and so on) flows through this extracellular liquid. As Alfred Pischinger asserted in *The Extracellular Matrix and Ground Regulation*, "Original seawater is the oldest system of communication between living cells."[3] As we shall see, this extracellular "marine plasma" contains a rich store of organic minerals and facilitates cellular conductivity by restoring the electrical potential of our cells. It creates the conditions for the optimal growth and development of the body's cells, a perfect nutrigenomic influence for achieving intracellular and extracellular homeostasis. When the extracellular fluid is different from its original oceanic origins, defective genes become activated. Nobel laureate Alexis Carrel (1873–1944) showed that cells can live almost indefinitely when they are kept in an optimum environment. As he stated in his Nobel lecture in 1912, "The cell is immortal. It is merely the fluid in which it floats that degenerates."[4]

This chapter is thus divided into two complementary sections, the intracellular fluid and the extracellular fluid.

INTRACELLULAR FLUID

Nutraceuticals are components of foods or dietary supplements with a medicinal or therapeutic effect. In general, they are taken in amounts higher than what can be obtained from the diet. Inadequate intake of several vitamins are associated with chronic disease.[5] For example, inadequate amounts of folate are associated with some cancers and birth defects. Folate and vitamins B_{12} and B_6 are required for homocysteine metabolism, a marker of inflammation and associated with coronary artery disease and Alzheimer's disease. Vitamin E and lycopene decrease the risk of prostate cancer. Vitamin D deficiency is associated with a host of illnesses, including heart disease, brain disease, osteoporosis, and fractures; these can be prevented by taking vitamin D and calcium.

There is much confusion about what supplements one should take. Instead of providing a long list of anti-inflammatory supplements, and since *WellMan* is about helping you develop a program to control inflammation, I believe it is more practical to focus on an overview of what you should supplement to optimize your well-being.

Ten Principals of Intracellular Health

1. Health and disease are determined by the vitality of the 60 trillion cells that make up our bodies and the various organs comprising them.

2. Nearly all diseases develop within organs at the cellular level. Inflammation is a major cause of most chronic disease.

3. Essential nutrients are needed for the thousands of biochemical reactions in each cell and to minimize the effects of inflammation.

4. The primary cause of cellular malfunction is a deficiency of vitamins, minerals, hormones, and other nutrients required for cell fuel.

5. Stress and aging (both mental and physical) will change the demand for nutrients required by the various cells of organs.

6. Nutrients are also required in different amounts as determined by an individual's genetic predisposition, lifestyle, and medical history.

7. Cardiovascular and neurological complications are the most prevalent of all ailments because those cells consume vitamins and other essential nutrients at higher rates than the cells of other organs.

8. Eternity Medicine Institutes, which provide a new context for health and many unique products, are the ideal sites to optimize both your intracellular and extracellular environment.

9. Dietary supplementation with enzymes, hormones, vitamins, and other nutrients is a key process in the prevention and treatment of cardiovascular conditions and other chronic diseases associated with imflam-aging.

10. Core nutraceuticals, containing antioxidants, enzymes, minerals, omega-3 fatty acids, and vitamins, should be consumed daily by all individuals. In addition, targeted nutraceuticals aimed at specific problems should also be taken to help support cell function while correcting cell malfunction in any diseased organs.

A Sample Supplement Plan

What follows is a fairly extensive supplement plan from one of our clients. Your program should contain at least some of the same nutraceuticals, since we know that our foods are being grown on nutrient-depleted soil and our health is suffering. Let us look at some of the nutrients taken by one of our WellMen, who has been on our program for more than a decade. In addition to core nutraceuticals and a full hormonal restoration program, he takes the following targeted supplements:

- Lycopene—Antioxidant, lowers blood pressure, prevents prostate cancer, and lowers LDL cholesterol.

- Indole-3-carbinol—Prevents development of estrogen-enhanced cancers.

- Resveratrol—Antioxidant, anti-inflammatory, increases nitric oxide and blood flow.

- Chondroitin sulfate—Large protein molecule found in cartilage, helps the pain of arthritis.

- Glucosamine—Main amino acid in connective tissue, helps transport sulfur into tissues.

- Green tea extract—Good antioxidant, helps the heart and brain, helps blood sugar and weight loss.

- Garlic (allicin)—Antibacterial, lowers LDL cholesterol, raises nitric oxide, lowers blood pressure, blood thinner.

- Boron—Aids vitamin D, decreases inflammation, regulates hormones, prevents prostate cancer, helps memory.

- Chromium picolinate—Regulates blood sugar, burns calories, increases HDL cholesterol, stimulates muscle and bone growth.

- Alpha-lipoic acid—Metal chelator, helps insulin levels, neutralizes free radicals, prevents cataracts, improves memory, protects collagen.

- Arginine—Builds muscle, enhances fat metabolism, increases growth hormone and nitric acid levels.

- Saw palmetto—Anti-inflammatory, protects the prostate, strengthens the immune system, helps male pattern baldness.

- Tryptophan—Precursor to serotonin, helps mood, and sleep, decreases appetite.

- D-Ribose—Low-glycemic sugar, helps energy production in heart and striated muscle.

- Bilberry—Helps eyesight, slows cataracts, reduces diabetic retinopathy, improves circulation, antibacterial.

- Pycnogenol—Mixture of antioxidants from pine tree, improves nitric oxide and circulation, anti-inflammatory, prevents cancer.

- Niacin (vitamin B3)—Decreases lipoprotein(a), lowers LDL cholesterol, raises HDL cholesterol, lowers triglycerides, decreases fibrinogen, helps adrenal glands.

- Probiotic—Increases friendly gut bacteria, improves immune factors and digestion, makes lactose.

- Evening primrose oil—Anti-inflammatory, helps you lose weight, lowers blood pressure, prevents clots, good source of GLA.

- Branched-chain amino acids (BCAAs; leucine, isoleucine, and valine)—Stimulates protein synthesis and decreases protein breakdown.

- Glutamine—Balances sugar, improves energy and memory, weight loss, promotes healthy acid-base balance, healthy gut.

- Oligomeric proanthocyanidins (OPCs)—Flavonoids and powerful antioxidants from grape seed extract, pine bark extract, and red wine extract.

- Curcumin (turmeric)—Anti-inflammatory, lowers LDL cholesterol, prevents cancer, helps cognition and inflammatory bowel disease.

- Carnitine—Made from lysine and methionine, energizes heart and brain, lowers LDL cholesterol and triglycerides, increases HDL cholesterol, increases oxygenation.

- L-Lysine—Helps the body produce antibodies, hormones, and enzymes, helps fight herpes, protects eye lenses.

Most of you will not take this rather rigorous supplement program. My advice is to individualize your own program. First, everyone should take core nutrients: multivitamins, Marine Plasma (minerals; see below), antioxidants (vitamins C and E, coenzyme Q_{10}, alpha-lipoic acid, glutathione), fish oil, probiotics, magnesium, vitamin D_3, and enzymes. Then, choose targeted nutrients depending on your genetic history, lifestyle, and medical history. Most nutraceuticals can be researched online at many excellent sites with extensive data. For example, if you go to the National Library of Medicine (Medline, www.pubmed.gov) and enter "omega-3s" you will find nearly 20,000 references. Many of these supplements have thousands of evidence-based research articles to support them. These are wonder nutrients that have multiple "side benefits" and, unlike most pharmaceuticals, have no side effects. I believe these nutrients are key to optimizing our health.

EXTRACELLULAR FLUID

The fluid that bathes each cell, known as the extracellular fluid, is a remnant of the ocean within each of us. Every cell in the body is connected through this fluid to our origins in the Earth's oceans. We, therefore, need great water and balanced micronutrients to optimize our extracellular fluid. Of all the items in our diet, the daily intake of water is the most important. Without it, we are unable to maintain the water balance of the body.

WATER GAINED	WATER LOST
Fluid	Urine (1,500 ml)
Food (water content)	Skin (900 ml)
Oxidation of hydrogen in food	Expired air (400 ml)
	Feces (200 ml)
Total ± 3 liters per day	*Total ± 3 liters per day*

More than 75 percent of Americans are chronically dehydrated, meaning we don't get the 8–10 servings of water each day (about 2 liters total) recommended by most health experts. Fluids like coffee, tea, alcohol, and juice do not count as water and can even dehydrate you more. For ideal health, you probably need to consume perhaps 2–3 times this amount.[6] A study published in the *Journal of the American Diabetic Association* showed that women who drink five glasses of water per day had 45 percent less risk of colon cancer.[7] Similar results have been seen for breast cancer. A survey of over 3,000 American adults at the New York Hospital at Cornell Medical Center indicates that 8–10 glasses of water a day could significantly reduce back and joint pain in up to 80 percent of sufferers. And lastly, German researchers recently showed that drinking just two glasses of water a day increased the metabolic rate a whopping 33 percent.[8]

Fereydoon Batmanghelidj, M.D., author of *Your Body's Many Cries for Water*, states that a whole host of diseases can be cured just by consuming more water. People are not sick, they are just thirsty, according to Dr. Batmanghelidj. "It is chronic water shortage in the body that causes most of the diseases of the human body."[9] The solution for prevention and treatment of those diseases is increased water intake on a regular basis.

Dr. Batmanghelidj shows that there are three stages of water regulation in the body in the different phases of life:

- Phase One—the stage of life of a fetus in the uterus of the mother.

- Phase Two—the phase of growth (anabolic) until full height and width is achieved (approximately age 18–25).

- Phase Three—the stage of life from fully grown to death (catabolic).

Because of a gradual failing of thirst sensation in the later decades, our body becomes chronically and increasingly dehydrated. The ratio of the volume of body water inside cells to the volume outside of cells changes from 1.1 to 0.8, which affects the efficiency of cell activity. Remember that water, the solvent of the body, regulates all functions, including the activity of the solutes it dissolves and circulates. Histamine and other transmitters (prostaglandins, kinins) become active to promote increased water intake. This excessive activity can cause allergies, asthma, and chronic pains in the body. Dyspeptic pain is the most important signal for the body denoting dehydration. It is also important to recognize that hunger often masks the need for water intake.

The human body is over 70 percent water and your blood is 90 percent water. Water is truly the source of life: the blood of the body is akin to the water of the earth. Most of us have about five liters of blood, all of which passes through the heart every three minutes (the heart beats 100,000 times per day, moving about eight tons each day). *Everything in our body responds to our blood and extracellular fluid*—this biological terrain (*milieu interieur*) is a microcosm of the sea itself. Most Americans have a very acidic biological terrain, which sets in motion a destructive cycle of imbalance, weight gain, and disease. This excess acid robs the blood of oxygen and metabolism slows. Food digests more slowly and tends to ferment, creating yeast and mold throughout the body. When you restore the quality of this internal "marine terrain" to its original form, every cell, organ, and tissue begins to respond and function as it was intended.

An Alkaline Lifestyle

By switching to a more alkaline lifestyle—by using LIV Water and more alkaline-forming foods—our blood is cleansed, we lose weight, and we become stronger, more energetic, and healthier. How is LIV Water different from the water most of us are familiar with? LIV Water's origins are based on the philosophy of Vicktor Schauberger (1885–1958), an Austrian scientist and visionary who pointed the way to a new understanding of water and natural energies.

After serving in World War One, Schauberger was employed by Prince Adolf Schaumburghippe, who gave him responsibility for 21,000 hectares of almost untouched forest land. He wrote: "I was drawn time and time again into the forest. I could sit for hours on end and watch the water flowing by without ever becoming tired or bored. Gradually, I began to play a game with water's secret powers; surrendering my free consciousness and allowing the water to take possession of it for a while. Little by little this game turned to a profoundly earnest venture, because I realized that one could detach one's own consciousness from the body and attach it to that of the water."[10]

He began to perceive water as the "earth's blood" and recognized that it must be allowed to flow along natural courses and kept at low temperature with the help of the forest shade if it was not to be spoiled. He noticed how water running from a mountain spring was at its greatest density, the so-called "anomaly point" at 4°C, and apparently at its highest quality. Salmon and trout during spawning drive themselves toward these sources, and the richest vegetation is found at these spots. One night during spawning time, Schauberger witnessed the following: "In the moonlight falling directly onto the crystal-clear water, every movement of the fish, gathered in large numbers, could be observed. Suddenly the trout dispersed, due to the appearance of a particularly large fish, which swam up from below to confront the waterfall. It seemed as if it wished to disturb the other trout and danced in great twisting movements in the undulating water, as it swam quickly to and fro. . . . I saw it fleetingly under a conically shaped stream of water, dancing in a wild spinning movement, the reason for which was at first not clear to me. It then came out of this spinning movement and floated motionlessly upwards. . . . There, in the fast flowing water, with a vigorous tail movement, it disappeared."[11]

Within the phenomenon, he saw evidence for his theory that the trout exploited some hitherto unknown source of energy within water. Unlike the scientists of today who see water as an inert substance, Schauberger saw water as a "living entity," with a structure and character, something that breathes and goes through the process of dying and renewal. Water can be healthy or unhealthy. Schauberger states, "Water is an organic magnet, and at the same time a transformer, a receiver, and a transmitter. It is the mediator or accumulator of growth, which mediates life."

LIV Water (SpaceAqua USA, www.spaceaqua.com) uses a machine capable of imitating nature to reproduce the physical hydrodynamic qualities of pure, natural spring water. It is thought that mimicking natural rhythmic whirlpools enhances the water's structure to its nanometric dimensions. I cannot stress enough how important it is to consume enough good water like LIV Water to optimize our health. It is best to consume water in the following manner:

- You should drink 1 liter every 2–3 hours.

- Drink most of your water between meals.

- Drink throughout the day; don't wait until you feel thirsty or hungry.

- Drink an extra liter for each hour of exercise.

The Internal Ocean

The link between blood and seawater was first hinted at by French biologist Claude Bernard (1813–1878), who formulated the concept of the "internal milieu" (internal terrain) and homeostasis. Bernard, a rival of Louis Pasteur, recognized that the body was largely water and that the internal milieu was a self-maintaining "marine environment."

It was, however, Rene Quinton (1866–1925), an ardent admirer of Bernard, who really sought to understand this internal environment and the process of sustaining it. He reasoned that if life evolved in a marine environment, and if, as Bernard proposed, health is contingent on maintaining and conserving a constant biochemical, electrolytic, and thermal milieu, then that milieu ought to be oceanic. Quinton found that the blood contained the same minerals and trace elements, in a similar proportion, as ocean water. He recognized that all organisms strive to maintain an interior milieu closely reflective of the original oceanic soup from which they evolved.

He studied waters obtained from massive plankton vortices, some hundreds of miles in diameter. He was convinced that the living waters obtained from these blooms, what he called "marine plasma," were analogous to mammalian plasma. In 1897, he set out to prove this at the Laboratory of Physiology, College de France. In a series of experiments, he drained nearly all the blood from living dogs and when these animals were on the verge of death, he infused cold-filtered, isotonic marine plasma. The dogs quickly recovered. These experiments ushered in the era of "marine therapy." Quinton and others advocated this marine plasma as a substitute for blood and helped save many soldiers lives during World War One. They also tried marine plasma for everything from cholera to tuberculosis.

The earth is a microcosm of our bodies. It is 70 percent water, as are our bodies; the pH of the ocean and our bodies should both be alkaline (7.35–7.45 pH), and the mineral ratio in our bodies mirrors that of the seas. The ocean is the amniotic fluid of the earth, containing the genetic blueprint that evolves all of life. Perhaps this is why the aging process does not occur in the seas as it does on land: a comparison between the cells of an adult whale and the cells of a newly born whale show no evidence of the changes we see when we look at adult and newborn land mammals. In addition, we do not find chronic disease in the ocean.

At the root of our food chain, servicing all the oceans, 320 million trillion gallons of water, are plankton blooms that seasonally arise in locations throughout the world's open oceans. These blooms are vortices that stir up the ocean floor, releasing nutrients and microbes that in turn seed the exponential growth of phytoplankton within the bloom. (This produces more vegetation than all land-based vegetation combined.) As phytoplankton populations explode, the larger zooplankton, such as krill, feed on the plankton and in turn digest and secrete a fluid that is packed with microbe-transformed crystalloid minerals, microenzymes, RNA, DNA, vitamins, and a host of marine co-factors. Fish lay their eggs in the bloom and whales travel thousands of miles to feed on the plankton and krill, protected by the virtual walls of the vortex acting as a great "marine nest." The rarefied water inside the bloom supports the entire oceanic food chain.

Quinton and his successors proved through over 100,000 case studies that marine plasma can play a significant role in healing and optimizing our well-being. At one time, the Quinton family funded free clinics throughout Europe and marine plasma was recognized as a pharmaceutical in the *Dictionnaire Vital* (France's equivalent to the *Physicians' Desk Reference*). The safety and efficacy of marine plasma has been shown in over 20,000 cases during the last forty years. Laboratory Quinton, located in Spain, uses the original plankton bloom off the coast of France and this water is available as Marine Plasma (Quinton America, www.plasmaquinton.com). The sterile ampules have been used to treat atopic dermatitis, chronic fatigue, and acute diarrhea, as well as for improving athletic performance. Marine Plasma appears to have powerful anti-inflammatory properties, which helps explain its many uses.

Most mineral supplements are composed of inorganic minerals that must be first converted by healthy "gut" bacteria in order to be absorbed. Much of that "rock" simply leaves the body as fast as it came in or, worse, sticks around congesting the internal organs. Plankton and microorganisms transform inorganic minerals found in the sea to their organic state, which is easily taken up by the intestine through passive diffusion. A complete spectrum of minerals is needed to metabolize the amino acids we consume, but the soil that grows our food no longer has many of these trace minerals we crave. We overeat in a futile attempt to restore this fundamental "organic" balance, but living off the land no longer provides the nutrients needed to maintain our internal ocean. Our land-locked bodies are nutritionally starved. Marine Plasma maintains an optimal internal environment (biological terrain) that is critical for health and longevity.

SUMMARY

- Advanced supplementation today is essential to optimize your health.

- Cells are immortal. It is the "fluid" in which they float that degenerates. Intracellular supplementation is only half the story; extracellular supplementation supplies the other key factor for health.

- Everyone should take "core" essential nutrients. Each person will also need to take "targeted" nutrients, depending on their genetic, lifestyle, and medical history.

- LIV Water has significant property differences compared to tap, bottled, and other machine-generated waters. It also has superior clinical advantages.

- It is essential that we maintain our "interior milieu," closely reflective of the original oceanic soup that we all evolved from. The aging process does not occur in the sea, but mammals do not do as well on land. It is important to restore our internal ocean.

- Marine Plasma has been shown to enhance athletic performance and improve a host of clinical conditions. It is the only living fluid on the planet that maintains the optimal internal environment critical for health and longevity.

CHAPTER 8

Lifelong (Mind-Body) Learning

Mind-body therapies not only improve overall health but also have a positive and measurable effect on specific conditions and diseases. Two key principles underpin the various therapies. First, the mind can affect the body in positive or harmful ways. Second, whatever you do physically has an impact on consciousness. A great deal of research reveals that psychological and spiritual practices, such as meditation, relaxation, guided imagery, and biofeedback, can have a useful impact on physical problems, including pain.

—KENNETH R. PELLETIER,
AUTHOR OF *MIND AS HEALER, MIND AS SLAYER*

THIS FINAL CHAPTER ON LIFELONG (mind-body) learning is divided into two parts. First, we discuss mind-body practices, which employ a variety of techniques designed to facilitate the mind's capacity to affect bodily function and symptoms. Second, everything we have ever known or felt or will feel is mental. Our entire perceived and imagined world is self-created within our head (our personal worldview). As medical doctors, we have come to recognize that the "ordering of consciousness" is as important to health as nutrition, exercise, supplements, hormones, and the lifestyle choices we make.

MIND-BODY PRACTICES

*Living and perceiving only through your head is why
life gets so confusing, stressful, and dry. Without enough
heart, you feel like you're living just to survive.
Through the heart you access more of your real spirit
and learn to become who you really are.*
—Doc Lew Childre, author of The HeartMath Solution

Mind-body medicine is a very old concept. Until about 300 years ago, virtually all philosophy and medicine treated the mind-body as an integral whole. The eighteenth century mechanistic and reductionist worldview led to the mind and body being separated.

The research that rediscovered the importance of mind-body medicine took place in 1974 at the Rochester School of Medicine and Dentistry, where psychologist Robert Ader showed that the immune systems of white rats had learned specific conditioned responses. Until this time, learning was thought to take place only in the brain and nervous system. Ader gave the rats a nausea-producing drug called cyclophosphamide to condition them to associate saccharine water with nausea and avoid it (classic Pavlovian conditioning). The problem was that many of the rats, although young and healthy, were getting sick and dying. Ader discovered that, in addition to causing nausea, cyclophosphamide was also lowering the number of T cells (which fight infection) in the immune system. Eventually, just giving the rats saccharine water alone (without cyclophosphamide) was all that it took to decrease T cells.[1] Classic conditioning had triggered a learned association with the taste of saccharine water and the suppression of T cells, which, in turn, made the rats more susceptible to disease and death. Until this experiment, the medical profession had believed that the central nervous system and the immune system were completely separate entities.

This research has been replicated many times since then, and the findings have given rise to a new field of mind-body medicine called psychoneuroimmunology (PNI). An explosion of PNI research has shown how our mind, beliefs, and emotions can profoundly affect physical well-being and our health.

Mutual Effects between the Mind and the Body

Mind-body interactions are not rare events but common occurrences in our everyday life. These interactions are mediated by nerves and hormones and act as an integrated whole.

Emotions—Emotions such as embarrassment cause physical responses such as blushing.

Stress Response—Stress and anxiety raise the levels of the hormones cortisol and epinephrine in the body. These have a variety of physical effects, including changes to the immune system, increased heart rate, and slowing of the digestive system.

Humor—Laughter has been shown to lower blood pressure, reduce levels of stress hormones, boost immunity (increasing T and B cells), and release endorphins (natural analgesics that produce a general sense of well-being).

Imagery—We can affect the way our body behaves just by using our imagination. For example, imagine unwrapping a chocolate. Feel the paper crinkling under your fingers, smell the aroma that is released, then imagine the taste and feel of it melting on your tongue. This imagery will no doubt have activated your salivary glands.

Exercise—Exercise has a variety of effects on the brain, including:

- Improved blood flow

- Release of endorphins, mood enhancers, and analgesics similar to morphine

- Alteration of serotonin levels in the brain

- Increased production of BDNF (brain-derived neurotrophic factor), a chemical that helps neurons grow and connect.

Massage and Physical Contact—Physical contact with another human (or an animal) can induce feelings of relaxation and well-being. Massage is a recognized agent for lowering stress.

Sex Hormones—Sex hormones (testosterone and estrogen) alter thoughts and behavior.

Posture—Studies have established that if we stand upright with head erect, smile, and breathe deeply, it is impossible to "feel" depressed.

Immune System—Immune molecules known as cytokines can initiate brain actions. Some cytokines help the brain recuperate by sending messages that set off a series of sickness responses, such as fever. The immune molecules also can trigger feelings of sluggishness, sleepiness, and loss of appetite, behaviors that encourage people to rest while they are ill.

Listening—Music can enhance mood and even have an analgesic effect by encouraging endorphin release. Biological sounds, such as a mother's heartbeat, have been used to lower infants' stress. Conversely, noise can increase heart rate, blood pressure, respiration rate, and blood cholesterol levels.

Breathing—By controlling breathing patterns, it is possible to reduce anxiety and stress responses.

The Efficacy of Mind-Body Therapies

Essential to integral health is the notion that the healing process does not work independently but relies on the changes in an individual's consciousness—behavior, attitude, worldview, environment, and lifestyle are all important. Emotional stress can cause inflammation just as easily as oxidized cholesterol. Many mind-body therapies help reduce inflammation and move the person toward health. There is now overwhelming research that a variety of mind-body practices can be very effective as adjuncts to conventional medicine for the treatment of many common clinical conditions:

- Coronary artery disease, high blood pressure, and strokes
- Insomnia
- General pain syndromes, fibromyalgia, and low-back pain
- Headaches
- Arthritis
- Cancer
- Recovery from surgery
- Asthma
- Chronic obstructive pulmonary disease
- Dermatological disorders
- Living with HIV
- Irritable bowel syndrome, peptic ulcers, and incontinence
- Tinnitus
- Pregnancy and labor

Specific Mind-Body Therapies

Here are a few of the more popular mind-body practices. Before consulting with one of these practitioners, make sure they are qualified and registered. Contact the relevant professional organizations for details and a list of practitioners in your area.

Meditation and Relaxation

Meditation is a long-standing feature of many spiritual traditions. Herbert Benson, M.D., and his research colleagues from Harvard University sought to elucidate the underlying science of meditation. He found four key elements central to the various meditative practices around the world and named this the "relaxation response."[2] These key elements include:

- A quiet environment without interruptions

- A mental device (a rhyme or mantra)

- A passive, accepting attitude

- An upright, yet relaxed posture

Research has shown that this therapy can lower blood pressure, relax muscles, and improve digestion and lung function in addition to other health benefits.

Guided Imagery

Guided imagery enlists the individual's imagination, together with relaxation, in evoking one or more of the senses—sound, vision, touch, or movement. Imagery is thus more than just visualization. Imagery is also related to hypnosis in that they both elicit similar states of consciousness. Research shows that imagery can reduce pain and anxiety, shorten hospital stays, reduce need for medication, and lessen side effects from treatment.

Hypnosis

In the eighteenth century, Franz Anton Mesmer (1734–1815) introduced this practice to medicine. The hypnotic state is similar to other forms of deep relaxation, with reduced sympathetic activity, decreased blood pressure, slowed heart rate and breathing, and altered brain wave activity. It is effective in gaining access to deeper levels of the mind in order to bring about changes in behavior. It can be used for analgesia in surgery, to control allergies, reduce stress, and help people stop smoking and lose weight.

Biofeedback

Biofeedback is a practice in which the individual learns to consciously regulate body functions such as heart rate, temperature, or blood pressure that are not normally accessible to voluntary control. Subjects are hooked up to a biofeedback machine that transmits signals about their breathing, muscles, heart rate, or brain wave functions. In this way, people gain a sense of control and learn to realize and achieve their desired outcome. With more sensitive feedback devices, treatment for incontinence, esophageal spasm, and stomach acidity has also been effective.[3]

Autogenic Training

Autogenic training is another useful technique to induce the relaxation response. It was developed in the 1930s by German psychiatrist Johannes Schultz. It includes actively focusing on feelings of warmth and heaviness in the limbs, with a passive focus on breathing to let it happen. Autogenic training can help various ailments, from stress and anxiety to high blood pressure and eczema.

Progressive Relaxation

Progressive relaxation was first described by American physician Edmund Jacobson in the 1920s. In this practice, you are taught to detect even the slightest muscle contraction as you scan your body from head to toe in order to achieve a deep degree of muscle relaxation. Progressive relaxation can help a variety of stress disorders, especially those that affect muscles, like tension headaches and fibromyalgia.

Gestalt Therapy

Gestalt therapy was developed by the German psychoanalyst Fritz Perls in the 1960s. Here, the person gains awareness of habitual thoughts, feelings, and actions and learns how to express any thoughts and emotions that may be repressed. The name comes from the German word for "organized whole."

Bioenergetics

Bioenergetics is similar to Gestalt therapy in that it is based on the belief that emotions are physically trapped within the body. It was originated in the 1950s by psychiatrist and psychoanalyst Wilhelm Reich (1897–1957) and expanded by psychotherapist Alexander Lowen, one of Reich's students.

Eye-Movement Desensitization and Reprocessing (EMDR)

EMDR was introduced by the American psychologist Francine Shapiro in 1987. It integrates elements of psychotherapy with eye movements. Certain types of eye movements are associated with stressful events. Therapy can help desensitize the client. EMDR has proven useful in treatment of traumatic disorders such as post-traumatic stress, phobias, and anxiety.[4]

Neurolinguistic Programming (NLP)

NLP was developed in the 1970s by psychotherapists John Grinder and Richard Bandler. An NLP practitioner helps a person consciously reprogram their patterns of speech and body language with the aim of improving their communication skills, bringing about personal change.

Rational Emotional Behavior Therapy (REBT)

Developed by American psychoanalyst Albert Ellis in 1955, the technique is designed to replace the irrational thinking behind negative emotions with more positive and flexible patterns of thought to help people attain their goals. It is useful for anxiety, stammering, depression, and addictions.

Freeze Frame

Freeze frame was developed by Doc Lew Childre from the Heart-Math Institute, in Boulder Creek, California. Learning how to "freeze frame" means understanding how to choose your perceptions of reality so they are the healthiest and most productive possible. Recordings of heart rate variability document the success of this treatment.[5]

OUR WORLDVIEW

> *Integral health is the process through which we humans achieve well-being by the ordering of consciousness. This includes the expansion of consciousness (knowledge) and the intensification of consciousness (wisdom).*
> —GRAHAM SIMPSON, M.D.

Humanity has evolved from simple consciousness to self-consciousness and is now ready for its next major transition, from self-consciousness to integral consciousness. Integral consciousness is an emergent psycho-historical development. With this awareness, the interaction between the physician and patient changes. We can no longer adhere to the mechanistic "doctor knows best," fix-it mentality that conventional medicine has upheld throughout much of the last century, treating symptoms of illness instead of getting to the root of a person's problem. Integral health is integrative, inclusive, comprehensive, and balanced. As Ken Wilber, founder of the Integral Institute, in Louisville, Colorado, writes, "To understand the whole, it is necessary to understand the parts. To understand the parts, it is necessary to understand the whole. Such is the circle of understanding."[6] A particular medical system will have a strong influence on the cultural worldview, which will set limits to individual awareness. We can go around these limits in any direction, because they are all mutually determining: they all cause, and are caused, by the others.

Knowledge is growing exponentially—in fact, knowledge is now believed to be doubling every two years. This has important implications for all of us. In order to make sense of the vast amount of knowledge coming our way, it essential to have a context that organizes this information to help enhance our consciousness and worldview. Historians, psychologists, philosophers, and others have each independently recognized that the mounting crisis for Western civilization is in fact the beginning of a fundamental restructuring of consciousness.

The Meta Story

The key idea is that consciousness has unfolded in five distinct stages or structures over time. Educator Page Smith, author of *Killing the Spirit*, described this as an "uneasy awareness," our dim knowledge of the human race's fascinating past. Smith further states that "without some knowledge of that past, a man or woman cannot be fully human, he or she cannot be truly a person at home in the world."[7]

One of the primary ways humans provide meaning is by telling stories. Joseph Campbell, author of *The Hero with a Thousand Faces* and many other books on mythology, spent his life uncovering the essential stories (myths) that humankind has used to inform their worldview and their actions. Campbell often wondered what the "new story" would be for us in the twenty-first century that would provide meaning and a sense of wholeness. We believe the new story is the story of the universe, a Meta Story that transcends all previous stories. It is made up of three distinct, related stories:

- The story of the cosmos (15 billion years)
- The story of the earth (5 billion years)
- The human story (5 million years)

Life is possible only because the universe is developing in the precise fashion it is. Life demands awareness and it is life that gives rise to consciousness. Here, we will focus on the human story.

THE STAGES OF CONSCIOUSNESS

	Time	Sense Organ	Awareness	Culture	Social	Spirit
Archaic	5 million– 200,000 B.C.	Body-kinesthetic	Visceral	Latent; Egoless	Nomadic hunters	Participation mystique
Magical	200,000– 10,000 B.C.	Ear	Emotional	Music/dance; Egoless	Hunter-gatherers	Ritual
Mythical	10,000– 2000 B.C.	Mouth	Imagination	Myth; Egoless	Farming; Language	Gods/ symbols
Mental	2000 B.C.– present	Eye	Reflection; Neocognition	Science Art; Egocentric	Industry; Fear/ alienation; Knowledge	God/ dogma
Integral	Future	Meta-sense	Individuation; Concretion/ verition	Integral; Science; Ego-free	Love/ wholeness; Wisdom	Overself/ transcendent

Modified from: Gebser, J. *The Ever Present Origin.* Athens, OH: Ohio University Press, 1985.

Archaic Human (5 million to 200,000 B.C.)

Homo habilis ("handy man") appeared about 2 million years ago and had a brain about half the size of our modern brain. Although language had not developed, they did make stone tools. This archaic human, although advanced beyond all prior evolutionary stages, is still undifferentiated from the surrounding world and has no sense of self and thus no existential fear. The sense organ that predominates is the body-kinesthetic sense. Protolanguage may have had its beginnings around the fire at night. As the only species to control fire (approximately 1.4 million years ago), humans likely used this newfound force as an opportunity to begin exploring their environment and the ever-recurring problems of food and shelter.

Magical Human (200,000–10,000 B.C.)

By 45,000 years ago, humans had spread over most of Africa, Europe, and Asia and numbered about 1 million. During this period, these hunter-gatherers increased in population and sophistication. More advanced use of tools, mime, and ritual were added. The voluntary expressive use of the face and voice to transmit emotion began in this mimetic-magical period but advanced significantly in the mythical period with the development of the larynx and the modern vocal apparatus. The magical human begins to awaken to personal finiteness and vulnerability. The ear is the predominant sense organ of the magical human.

Mythical Human (10,000–2,000 B.C.)

The Neolithic age (New Stone Age) began about 10,000 years ago. Neolithic people differentiated themselves from all previous humans by settling in permanent villages. This was the result of two important developments: the growth of agriculture and the later taming of several kinds of animals. By 8000 B.C., most of the major institutions of humankind were established. Language is the hallmark of the mythical human, although no one knows how rapidly speech spread. The most elevated use of language in tribal societies is that of mythic invention, the myth being the prototypical integrative mind tool. The mouth is the dominant sense organ of this mythical human.

Mythic culture tends toward the rapid integration of knowledge. Myth governs the collective mind and a sense of "we" membership prevails. The mythic human is still egoless, lives in a dream state, and uses speech to tell stories that explain reality. Language allowed for the integration of knowledge, symbols, imagination, ideals, morality, and belief systems. With this expanded consciousness and the ability to more clearly picture the future, humankind needed to see this unfolding future as a promise that death was in the distance.

Mental Human (2,000 B.C.–Present)

A subtle change occurred in our worldview as we moved from the earlier magical-mythical worldview, with its cyclical sense of time, toward our modern linear time. A new and heightened awareness/fear of death followed as a direct result of farming and language. Fear can only exist in linear time and stubbornly sits at the center of our modern worldview.

Early Mental Human (2000 B.C. to A.D. 1500)—History, in the form of recorded events, began with the development of writing in this period. According to ancient Greek scholar Bruno Snell in *The Discovery of Mind*, Homer's characters use their eyes to see or to receive optical impressions. However, they apparently took no interest in the objective essence of sight. There was no word for perspective—as far as they were concerned it did not exist.[8]

The period of Western civilization following the collapse of the Roman Empire, from 500 to 1500 A.D., is called the Middle or Dark Ages. As Darcy Ribeiro writes, "The history of man in these last centuries is principally the history of the expansion of Western Europe which, constituting the nucleus of a new civilization, proceeded to launch itself on all people in successive waves of violence and oppression. In this movement, the whole world was shaken up and rearranged according to European design and in conformity with European interests. Each people, even each human being, was affected and caught up in the European economic system or in the ideals of power, justice, or politics inspired by it."[9]

Late Mental Human (1500 to present)—The beginning of the modern mental structure around 1500 A.D. was the result of four major actions that changed the course of humankind:

- World exploration that begin in the late 1400s

- The development of perspective and scientific inquiry

- The flow of inventions such as Gutenberg's movable type

- Industrial production, which began in earnest in the 1600s

The mental human relies on the eye for perceiving the world. This seeing and conceptualizing are commensurate with our mental reflective structure. How we see becomes an expression of our understanding of our world. Italian painter Giotto (circa 1267 to 1337) was the first artist of record to understand intuitively the benefits of painting a scene as if viewed from a stationary single point. The flat picture presentation, which was prevalent for a thousand years, acquired a third dimension of depth when Giotto's protoper-

Gebser's Scheme Underlies All Our Institutions

INSTITUTION	AUTHOR	ARCHAIC	MAGICAL	MYTHICAL	MENTAL	INTEGRAL
Art	Jean Gebser	None	Pre-perspectival	Un-perspectival	Perspectival	Aperspectival
War	Carl Von Clausewitz	No War	Tribal war	Political war	Eschatological war	Obsolete
Religion	Joseph Campbell	None	Ritual (totemism)	Gods (symbols)	God (dogma)	Transcendent
Education	Howard Gardner	Bodily intelligence	Musical intelligence	Linguistic intelligence	Spatial intelligence	Nature intelligence
Medicine	Larry Dossey	Wise women	Shaman	Thoth	ERA I and II medicine	Non-local mind (ERA 111)
Politics	Eric Voeglin	Experience of participation	Tribal organization	Cosmological Myth	Gnosticism-modernity	Flowing presence
Language	Merlin Donald	Episodic	Mimetic	Mythic	Theoretic	Meta-linguistic
Economics	E.F. Schumacher	None	Trade	Dual economy	Market economy	Meta-economy
Sociology	Bruce Mazlish	Clan	Tribe	Paternal landlord	Industrial cash nexus	Many stranded web
Technology	James Burke	Axes	Bows	Farming	Science	Infomatics
Psychology	Carl Jung	Sensing	Intuiting	Feeling	Thinking	Transcending
Ecology	Brian Swimme	Human emergence	Neolithic settlements	Classical civilization	Rise of nations	Ecozoic age

spective placed the viewer in front of the canvas. As significant as Giotto was, Filippo Brunelleschi (1377–1446), an Italian architect, is credited with the true discovery of Western linear perspective.

Thus, in addition to the notion of linear time, the mental human is now faced with perspective and the conquering of space. Besides illuminating space, perspective lends humans a sense of their own visibility and provides a sense of distance between human and objects. The conception of human as subject is based on a conception of world as object.

Early human's lack of spatial awareness is attended by a lack of ego. In order to objectify and qualify space, a self-conscious "I" is required that is able to stand opposite and confront space. Thus, from this time onward, humankind can be considered to have a self-consciousness rather than the simple consciousness of earlier periods. This is visible in a variety of ways: in the appearance of words expressing awareness and self-awareness in the Anglo-Saxon language, in the creation of the first novel, and in the emergence of a free-floating anxiety and fear of death that so affects the modern man.

Integral Human (Our Future)

Near the close of the nineteenth century, another new appreciation of space and time emerged. Pablo Picasso (1881–1973) and Georges Braque (1882–1963) invented a revolutionary new art form called cubism at the turn of the century. Cubism, in fact, embodied the first new way to perceive space since the time of Euclid, the father of geometry, 2,200 years earlier. Shortly after this time, Albert Einstein (1879–1955) overturned the foundations of classical physics with his theory of relativity, and physicists abandoned forever the notion of absolute space and time—the aperspectival worldview (space free and time free) had been born. A new "asperspectival" view is necessary for us if we are to look at the world and see it whole. Whereas the understanding of the mental structure depended on the concretion of space, our emerging epoch depends on the concretion of time. Only where time emerges as pure present and is no longer divided into its three phases of past, present, and future will it be concrete.

Eternity Medicine

In Howard Gardner's book *Five Minds for the Future*, the noted Harvard psychologist defines the five cognitive abilities that he believes will command a premium in the years ahead—the disciplinary mind, the synthesizing mind, the creating mind, the respectful mind, and the ethical mind. Nobel Prize–winning physicist Murray Gell-Mann (born 1929) believes that the mind most at a premium in the twenty-first century will be the mind that can synthesize well. The ability to put together information from disparate sources into a coherent whole is vital for lifelong learning, as we crave coherence and integration.

Another important insight is the fact that not only has our species gone through this evolutionary development but each one of us goes through our own psycho-historical development, remembering our own structures—sensing, intuiting, feeling, and thinking enables the integration and individuation of each of us so that the human personality becomes transparent to itself, enabling the spiritual to be directly aware. This is what John Eccles (1903–1997), winner of the Nobel Prize in Physiology or Medicine in 1963, suggests when he writes, "We have to recognize that we are spiritual beings with souls existing in a spiritual world as well as material beings with bodies and brains existing in a material world."[10]

We are truly in a unique position—knowledge is doubling every two years but technology now allows each of us to access the world's knowledge (the expansion of consciousness). We can also intensify consciousness (wisdom) and "experience" the emerging integral structure of consciousness that is space free and time free. This integral structure is real and does not concede anything to the supernatural. It is primarily through this integral structure that the spiritual can be directly experienced.

Just as the novel understanding of space gave birth to self-consciousness, a new understanding of time is now giving birth to the integral structure of consciousness. Space-free and time-free mind is unbounded and infinite in space and time, thus omnipresent, eternal, and ultimately one. We have begun to see evidence of the application of this changing worldview in a new spectrum of non-local healing.

SPECTRUM OF NON-LOCAL HEALING

Interacting Systems	Evidence of Interaction	Expression of Interaction
Humans and humans	Humans interact with each other non-locally—at a distance, without benefit of sensory- or energy-based exchanges of information. Many controlled studies deal with distant/intercessory prayer and other types of distant mental intent.[13] Hundreds of telesomatic events have been reported. Numerous controlled studies have documented nonlocal forms of gaining or conveying information (clairvoyance or telepathy).	Love, empathy, compassion, caring, unity, collective consciousness, the Universal or One Mind, God ("God is love"), Goddess, Allah, Tao, the Absolute
Humans and animals	Scores of studies involving various types of distance healing intent have been done using higher animals as "targets." These studies often involve prayer or "bio-PK" (psychokinesis).[12] Lost pets return to owners across vast distances to places they have never been.	Love, Empathy
Humans and living organisms	Scores of controlled studies have dealt with the distance effects of prayer and other types of positive distant healing intent. in which various "lower organisms" —bacteria, fungi, yeasts—are the targets, as well as seeds, plants, and cells of various sorts.	Love, Empathy
Humans and complex machines	Humans can mentally influence the behavior of sophisticated electronic biofeedback devices—affirmed by the collective record of more than 30 years of biofeedback research in hundreds of laboratories.[11] Humans also can mentally influence random event generators and other electronic instruments at a distance, as demonstrated in studies conducted at the Princeton Engineering Anomalies Research (PEAR) lab and many other institutions.	"Becoming one" or "falling in love" with the machine, interconnection, unity

SPECTRUM OF NON-LOCAL HEALING (continued)

INTERACTING SYSTEMS	EVIDENCE OF INTERACTION	EXPRESSION OF INTERACTION
Humans and simple machines	Humans can interact with and influence the behavior of freely swinging pendulums, mechanical cascade devices, and other relatively simple apparatuses, at a distance—affirmed by studies conducted at the PEAR lab and elsewhere.	"Becoming one" or "falling in love" with the machine, interconnection, unity
Complex physical devices/ systems	According to commonly accepted principles in physics, coupled harmonic oscillators, all common musical instruments and radio and television circuitry interact and resonate with each other. In general, all manner of physical systems—whether mechanical, electromagnetic, fluid, dynamical, quantum mechanical, or nuclear—display synergistically interactive vibrations with similar systems or with their environment.	Sympathetic or harmonic resonance
Subatomic particles	Subatomic particles such as electrons, once in contact, demonstrate simultaneous change—no matter how far apart—to the same degree. Bell's theorem, the Aspect experiment, and many other developments affirm these possibilities at the quantum-mechanical level.	Nonlocally correlated behavior, rudimentary or proto-love?

It is vital that the integral physician helps each person reorder their worldview to help realize that they exist within a process of space-time, not as isolated entities adrift in linear time. It is time to impart this knowledge of the interconnectedness of all life and how the spiritual flowing present can be deeply felt and experienced. To the extent we accomplish this task, we are truly healers. With a single, subtle voice, science, art, and the great spiritual traditions all communicate this notion today—that each of us is infinite, immortal, and indestructible.

SUMMARY

- Whatever you do physically has an impact on consciousness. Likewise, every thought registers a physical effect on the body.

- Consciousness has evolved in our species in five distinct stages or structures of consciousness over time, and each of us has gone through the same psycho-historical stages of development ("ontogeny recapitulates phylogeny").

- Humanity has evolved from simple consciousness to self-consciousness and we are now ready for the next transition from self-consciousness to integral consciousness (an emergent psycho-historical development).

- By recognizing and integrating our structures of consciousness, we develop "integral" consciousness. We become transparent to the transcendent (experience transcends faith).

- All (mind-body) learning needs to include a context for the integration of the psycho-historical development of our structures of consciousness. Integral health is the process through which humans achieve well-being by this ordering of consciousness.

- We have to recognize that we are spiritual beings with souls existing in a spiritual world as well as material beings with bodies and brains existing in a material world.

- Each of us is infinite, immortal, and indestructible.

Conclusion

As many of you now know, modern medicine has little to offer us in terms of health restoration for the most common causes of disease and disability in industrialized societies. Heart disease, which kills more than 50 percent, is a typical example. Once we recognize that "silent inflammation" is the primary cause of vascular disease and most other chronic disease, we can halt and even reverse this process.

Our modern Western diet is at the center of most of this disease. Our diet is so artificially concentrated with trans-fats, oils, sugar, and other refined carbohydrates that we are dying from excess rather than any deficiencies. This modern day affluence has to be reckoned with if we want to regain our health.

Toxin reduction and exercise are also important to restoring our health. Rest and sleep are vital: the average adult in the U.S. now sleeps less than seven hours and is sleep deprived for much of his or her life.

There are many non-invasive aesthetic procedures that will help a man "look good" as well as feel good. Restoration of hormones and advanced supplementation are key to optimizing our total health. It is essential for the modern man to pay attention to the water and minerals he takes in, for restoring the "ocean within" and helping to slow the aging process

Finally, our worldview has everything to do with our well-being.

Lifelong learning in the digital age will ultimately transform health-care. I believe that "consciousness" will replace the germ theory as part of the new green medicine that is emerging.

With the Integral Health Program outlined in *WellMan*, you have all the tools to regain optimum health and come to the realization that you are indeed infinite, immortal, and indestructible.

Resources

Chapter 1: Inflammation Control

Graham Simpson, M.D.
Eternity Medicine Institute
8930 W. Sunset Road, Suite 100
Las Vegas, NV 89148
(702) 248-4364
www.eternitymedicine.com
www.inflamaging.com

Chapter 2: Nutrition

Loren Cordain Ph.D.
Dept. of Health and Exercise
  Science
Colorado State University
Fort Collins, CO 80523
(970) 491-7436
www.thepaleodiet.com

Dr. Jon Roxarzade
The Eternity Diet
54 North Pecos Road, Suite C
Henderson, NV 89074
(702) 696-1000
www.eternitymedicine.com

Chapter 3: Toxin Reduction

Roni De Luz, Ph.D.
Vineyard Holistic Retreat
209 Franklin Street
Vineyard Haven, MA 02568
(508) 693-0001
www.mvholisticretreat.com

Dr. Alan Goldhammer
True North Health Center
1551 Pacific Avenue
Santa Rosa, CA 95404
(707) 586-5555
www.healthpromoting.com

Chapter 4: Exercise

Snap Fitness, Inc.
2411 Galpin Ct., Suite 110
Chanhassen, MN 55317
(952) 567-5992
www.snapfitness.com

Kersh Risk Management
2700 Research Drive, Suite 200
Plano, TX 75074
(800) 467-3005
www.kershwellness.com

Chapter 5: Graded Aesthetic Enhancement

Ageless Zone Medical Spa
  & Salon
5060 Meadowood Mall Circle
Reno, NV 89502
(775) 826-8888
www.agelesszonereno.com

Beautiful Forever Consulting
  Firm, Inc.
560 Sylvan Avenue
Englewood Cliffs, NJ 07632
(877) 772-6334
www.beautifulforever.com

Joseph Williams, M.D.
Advanced Medical Hair Institute
8945 Russel Road, #320
Las Vegas, NV 89148
(702) 257-0888
www.need-hair.com

Chapter 6: Restore Bio-Identical Hormones

Heart Check America
7690 West Sahara Avenue
Las Vegas, NV 89117
(702) 485-4673
(800) NEW-TEST (639-8378)

Jacob Rosenstein, M.D.
800 W. Arbrook, Suite 150
Arlington, TX 76015
(817) 467-5551
www.ntneurosurgery.com

Eternity Medicine Institute
8930 W. Sunset Road, Suite 100
Las Vegas, NV 89148
(702) 248-4364
www.eternitymedicine.com

Chapter 7: Advanced Supplementation

AnazaoHealth Corporation
6630 W. Arby Avenue, Suite 102
Las Vegas, NV 89118
(800) 723-7455
www.anazaohealth.com

LIV Water
2390 Overlook Court
Reno, NV 89509
(775) 240-7878
www.spaceaqua.com

Original Quinton—North
  America, Inc.
6900 Aragon Circle
Buena Park, CA 90620
(888) 278-4686
www.originalquinton.com

Chapter 8: Lifelong (Mind-Body) Learning

Integral Spirituality
P.O. Box 1508
Sausalito, CA 94966
(415) 332-2301
www.integrativespirituality.org

Or:

480 Gate 5 Road, Suite 246
Sausalito, CA 94965
(415) 331-1395

Eternity Medicine Institute
8930 W. Sunset Road, Suite 100
Las Vegas, NV 89148
(702) 248-4364
www.eternitymedicine.com

ETERNITY MEDICINE INSTITUTE LOCATIONS

For an Institute located in the U.S. or Internationally, please contact the Eternity Medicine Institute Corporate office at:

8930 W. Sunset Road, Suite 100
Las Vegas, NV 89148
Phone: (702) 248-4364 • Fax: (702) 248-1274
Toll-free: (888) 406-6462
www.eternitymedicine.com

HSA/HDHP INSURANCE OPTION

NPI Group has partnered with United Healthcare to provide an alternative to pay for EMI Age Management programs. For information on this great tax advantage option, contact:

Jennifer L. Pyle, Broker Consultant
NPI Group, LLC.
1588 Rio Grande Drive
Reno, NV 89521
(775) 622-1739   Office
(775) 201-9678   Fax
(775) 379-5309   Cell
jpyle@npinsgroup.com
www.npinsgroup.com

Dori Stone, Broker Consultant
NPI Group, LLC.
1588 Rio Grande Drive
Reno, NV 89521
(775) 622-1739   Office
(775) 201-9678   Fax
(775) 750-0115   Cell
dstone@npinsgroup.com
www.npinsgroup.com

AGE MANAGEMENT DIAGNOSTIC SERVICES

Age Diagnostic Laboratories
852 South Military Trail
Deerfield Beach, FL 33442
(877) 983-7863   Office
(866) 454-9650   Fax
www.adltests.com

Heart Check America
7690 West Sahara Avenue
Las Vegas, NV 89117
(702) 489-6305   Office
(702) 485-4098   Fax
(800) NEW-TEST (639-8378)
www.heartcheckamerica.com

HeartSmart Technologies
19700 Fairchild, Suite 300
Irvine, CA 92612
(949) 724.1700
www.heartsmartimt.com

References

Chapter 1: Inflammation Control

1. DeBusk, L.M., Y. Chen, T. Nishishita, et al. "Tie2 Receptor Tyrosine Kinase, a Major Mediator of Tumor Necrosis Factor Alpha–induced Angiogenesis in Rheumatoid Arthritis." *Arthritis Rheum* 48:9 (2003): 2461–2471.

2. Jeppeson, J., H.O. Hein, P. Suadicani, et al. "Low Triglycerides–High High-density Lipoprotein Cholesterol and Risk of Ischemic Heart Disease." *Arch Intern Med* 161:3 (2001): 361–366.

3. Ridker, P.M., R.J. Glynn, C.H. Hennekens "C-reactive Protein Adds to the Predictive Value of Total and HDL Cholesterol in Determining Risk of First Myocardial Infraction." *Circulation* 97:20 (1998): 2007–2011.

4. Lovejoy, H.B., Z.G. Bell Jr., T.R. Vizena. "Mercury Exposure Evaluations and Their Correlation with Urine Mercury Excavation. 4. Elimination of Mercury by Sweating." *J Occup Med* 15:7 (1973): 590–591.

5. Saloren, J.T., K. Seppänen, K. Nyyssönen, et al. "Intake of Mercury from Fish, Lipid Peroxidation, and the Risk of Myocardial Infarction and Coronary, Cardiovascular, and Any Death in Eastern Finnish Men." *Circulation* 91:3 (1995): 645–655.

6. Kajunder, E.O., and N. Ciftçioglu. "Nanobacteria: An Alternative Mechanism for Pathogenic Intra- and Extra-cellular Calcification and Stone Formation." *Proc Natl Acad Sci* 95:14 (1998): 8274–8279.

7. Ibid.

8. Loesche, W.J. "Periodontal Disease: Link to Cardiovascular Disease." *Compend Contin Educ Dent* 21:6 (2000): 463–466.

9. Sinatra, S. "Stay in the Sinatra-Smart Zone for Optimum Health." *The Sinatra Health Report* (May 2003).

10. Seshadri, S., A. Beiser, J. Selhub, et al. "Plasma Homocysteine as a Risk Factor for Dementia and Alzheimer's Disease." *New Engl J Med* 346:7 (2002): 476–483.

11. Danesh, J., R. Collins, R. Peto. "Lipoprotein(a) and Coronary Artery Disease. Meta-analysis of Prospective Studies." *Circulation* 102:10 (2000): 1082–1085.

12. Taubes, Gary. *Good Calories, Bad Calories.* New York: Anchor, 2008.

13. Putnam, J.J., et al. "Sugar and Starch Consumption Over the Twentieth Century." Washington, DC: United States Department of Agriculture (USDA) Economic Research Service, 2000.

14. Montori, V.M., A. Farmer, P.C. Wollan, et al. "Fish Oil Supplementation in Type 2 Diabetes: A Quantitative Systemic Review." *Diabetes Care* 23:9 (2000): 1407–1415.

15. Sears, Barry. *The Anti-Inflammation Zone.* New York: Collins Living, 2005.

16. Ford, E.S, W.H. Giles, W.H. Dietz. "Prevalence of the Metabolic Syndrome among U.S. Adults: Findings from the Third National Health and Nutrition Examination Survey." *JAMA* 287:3 (2002): 356–359.

17. Sears, Barry. *Toxic Fat.* Nashville, TN: Thomas Nelson, 2008.

18. Lundholm, K., G. Holm, T. Scherstén. "Insulin Resistance in Patients with Cancer." *Cancer Res* 38:12 (1978): 4665–4670.

19. Doll, R., and R. Peto. "The Causes of Cancer: Quantitative Estimates of Avoidable Risks of Cancer in the United States Today." *J Natl Cancer Inst* 66:6 (June 1981): 1191–1308.

20. Sears, Barry. Personal communication.

21. Aisen, P.S. "Anti-inflammatory Therapy for Alzheimer's Disease." *Neurobiol Aging* 21:3 (2000): 447–448.

22. Burgess, J.R., L. Stevens, W. Zhang, et al. "Long-Chain Polyunsaturated Fatty Acids in Children with Attention-Deficit Hyperactivity Disorder." *Am J Clin Nutr* 71:1 Suppl (2000): 327S–330S.

23. Stoll, A.L., W.E. Severus, M.P. Freeman, et al. "Omega-3 Fatty Acids in Bipolar Disorder: A Preliminary Double-blind Placebo-controlled Trial." *Arch Gen Psychiatry* 56:5 (1999): 407–412.

24. Peet, M., J.D. Laugharne, J. Mellor, et al. "Essential Fatty Acid Deficiency in Erythrocyte Membranes from Chronic Schizophrenic Patients and the Clinical Effects of Dietary Supplementation." *Prostaglandins Leukot Essent Fatty Acids* 55:1–2 (1996): 71–75.

25. Taubes, Gary. *Good Calories, Bad Calories.* New York: Anchor, 2008.

26. Willett, Walter. *Eat, Drink and Be Healthy.* New York: Simon & Schuster, 2002.

27. Simpson, Graham. *Spa Medicine*. North Bergen, NJ: Basic Health, 2004.

28. Pascot, A., J.P. Després, I. Lemieux, et al. "Contribution of Visceral Obesity to the Deterioration of the Metabolic Risk Profile in Men with Impaired Glucose Tolerance." *Diabetologia* 43:9 (2000): 1126–1135.

29. Cordain, Lauren. *The Paleo Diet*. New York: John Wiley and Sons, 2002.

30. de Lorgeril, M., P. Salen, J-L. Martin, et al. "Mediterranean Diet, Traditional Risk Factors, and the Rate of Cardiovascular Complications after Myocardial Infarction: Final Report of the Lyon Diet Heart Study." *Circulation* 99 (1999): 779–785.

31. Sears, Barry. *The Anti-Inflammation Zone*. New York: Collins Living, 2005.

Chapter 2: Nutrition

1. Steinberg, D. "Thematic Review Series: The Pathogenesis of Atherosclerosis. An Interpretive History of the Cholesterol Controversy: Part II: The Early Evidence Linking Hypercholesterolemia to Coronary Disease in Humans." *J Lipid Res* 46:2 (2005): 179–190.

Castelli, W.P., J.T. Doyle, T. Gordon, et al. "HDL Cholesterol and Other Lipids in Coronary Heart Disease. The Cooperative Lipoprotein Phenotyping Study." *Circulation* 55 (1977): 767-772.

3. Keys, A. "Coronary Heart Disease in Seven Countries." *Circulation* 41:4 Suppl (April 1970): 1–211.

4. Goslin, E.P. "Arteriosclerosis and Diabetes." *Ann Clin Med* 5 (1927): 1061–1079.

5. Stout, R.W. "Insulin-stimulated Lipogenesis in Arterial Tissue in Relation to Diabetes and Atheroma." *Lancet* 2:7570 (1968): 702–703.

6. Thorpe, G.L. "Treating Overweight Patients." *JAMA* 165:11 (1957): 1361–1365.

7. Pennington, A. *N Engl J Med* (1953).

8. Eaton, S.B. "Humans, Lipids and Evolution." *Lipids* 27:10 (1992): 814–820.

9. O'Keefe Jr., J., and L. Cordain. "Cardiovascular Disease Resulting from a Diet and Lifestyle at Odds with Our Paleolithic Genome: How to Become a 21st-Century Hunter-Gatherer." *Mayo Clin Proc* 79:1 (2004): 101–108.

10. Simopoulos, Artemis. *The Omega Diet*. New York: Collins Living, 1999.

11. de Lorgeril, M., P. Salen, J-L. Martin, et al. "Mediterranean Diet, Traditional Risk Factors, and the Rate of Cardiovascular Complications after Myocardial Infarction: Final Report of the Lyon Diet Heart Study." *Circulation* 99 (1999): 779–785.

12. [No authors listed.] "Dietary Supplementation with n-3 Polyunsaturated

Fatty Acids and Vitamin E after Myocardial Infarction: Results of the GISSI-Prevenzione Trial. Gruppo Italiano per lo Studio della Sopravvivenza nell'Infarto Miocardico." *Lancet* 354:9177 (1999): 447–455.

13. O'Keefe Jr., J., and L. Cordain. "Cardiovascular Disease Resulting from a Diet and Lifestyle at Odds with Our Paleolithic Genome: How to Become a 21st-Century Hunter-Gatherer." *Mayo Clin Proc* 79:1 (2004): 101–108.

14. Ibid.

15. Ibid.

16. Taubes, Gary. *Good Calories, Bad Calories.* New York: Anchor, 2008.

17. Nicolaïdis, S. "Early Systemic Responses to Orogastric Stimulation in the Regulation of Food and Water Balance: Functional and Electrophysiological Data." *Ann NY Acad Sci* 157:2 (1969): 1176–1203.

18. Center for Science in the Public Interest. "Liquid Candy." Available online at: http//www.cspinet.org/sodapop/liquid_candy.htm. Curhan, C., W.C. Willett, E.B. Rimm, et al. "Prospective Study of Beverage Use and the Risk of Kidney Stones." *Am J Epidemiol* 143:3 (1996): 240–247.

19. *Intl J Obesity* (July 2007).

20. Lutsey, P.L., L.M. Steffen, J. Stevens. "Dietary Intake and the Development of the Metabolic Syndrome: The Atherosclerosis Risk in Communities Study." *Circulation* 117:6 (February 2008): 754–761.

Chapter 3: Toxin Reduction

1. Watson, Brenda. *The Detox Strategy.* New York: Simon & Schuster, 2008.

2. Kolpin, D.W., E.T. Furlong, M.T. Meyer, et al. "Pharmaceuticals, Hormones, and Other Organic Wastewater Contaminants in U.S. Streams, 1999–2000: A National Reconnaissance." *Environ Sci Technol* 36:6 (2002): 1202–1211.

3. Groves, Barry. *Fluoride: Drinking Ourselves to Death.* Dublin, Ireland: Newleaf, 2002.

4. U.S. Environmental Protection Agency Pesticide Programs, 2002.

5. Rogers, Sherry. *Detoxify or Die.* New York: Prestige, 2002.

6. Environmental Working Group (EWG). "Bisphenol A: Toxic Plastics Chemical in Canned Food." Washington, DC: EWG, 2007. Available online at: www.ewg.org/reports/bisphenola.

7. Breiner, Mark A., D.D.S. *Whole-Body Dentistry.* Trumbull, CT: Quantum Health, 1999.

8. Rogers, Sherry. *Tired or Toxic? A Blueprint for Health.* New York: Prestige, 1990.

9. Environmental Working Group (EWG). The Human Toxome Project. www. ewg.org/sites/humantoxome/.

10. Watson, Brenda. *The Detox Strategy*. New York: Simon & Schuster, 2008.

11. Pelletier, C., P. Imbeault, A. Tremblay. "Energy Balance and Pollution by Organochlorines and Polychlorinated Biphenyls." *Obes Rev* 4:1 (2003): 17–24.

12. Krimsky, Sheldon. *Hormonal Chaos: The Scientific and Social Origins of the Environmental Endocrine Hypothesis*. Baltimore: Johns Hopkins University Press, 2002.

Chapter 4: Exercise

1. President Council on Physical Fitness and Sports. "Definitions: Health, Fitness, and Physical Activity." Accessed April 2010. www.fitness.gov/digest_mar2000.htm.

2. Paffenbarger R, Kambert I, et al. "Changes in Physical Activity and Other Lifeway Patterns Influencing Longevity." *Med Sci Sports Exercise*. 1994; 26(7):857–865.

3. Mayo Clinic. "Exercise: & Benefits of Healthy Activity." July 2009. Accessed April 2010 www.mayoclinic.com/health/exercise/HQ01676.

4. McHill HC., McMahan CA, et al. "Effects of Nonlipid Risk Factors on Atherosclerosis in Youth with a Favorable Lipoprotein Profile." *Circulation*. 2001; 103:1546–1550.

5. American College of Sports Medicine. *ACSM's Resource Manual for Guidelines for Exercise Testing and Prescription: Sixth Edition*. Baltimore: Wolters Kluwer: 2010.

6. Gallagher et al. *Am J Clin Nut*. 2000; 72:694–701.

7. National Institutes of Health. "Aim for a Healthy Weight." Accessed April 2010. www.nhlbisupport.com/bmi/bminojs.htm

8 Centers for Disease Control and Prevention. "About BMI for Adults." Accessed April 2010. www.cdc.gov/healthyweight/assessing/bmi/adult_ bmi/index.html.

9. Wolinsky I, Driskell J. *Sports Nutrition: Energy Metabolism & Exercise*. Boca Raton: CRC Press, 1998.

10. Association for Applied Sport Psychology. "Psychological Benefits of Exercise." Accessed April 2010. http://appliedsportpsych.org/Resource-Center/health-and-fitness/articles/psych-benefits-of-exercise.

11. Weyerer S, HupferB. "Physical Exercise and Psychological Health." *Sports Med*. 1994; 17(2):108–116.

12. Saltin B, Astrand P. "Free Fatty Acids and Exercise." *Am J Clin Nutr*. 1993; 57(5):752S–757S.

13. Ray US, Mukhopadhyaya S, et al. "Effect of Yogic Exercises on Physical and Mental Health of Young Fellowship Course Trainees." *Indian J Physiol Pharmacol.* 2001 Jan;45(1):37–53.

14. American Heart Association. "Exercise and Fitness." October 2009. Accessed April 2010. www.americanheart.org/presenter.jhtml?identifier= 1200013.

15. Bemben MG, Miccalip GA. "Strength and Power Relationships as a Function of Age." *J of Strength and Conditioning Research.* 1999; 13:330–338.

16. Whaley MH, Kampert JB, et al. "Physical Fitness and Clustering of Risk Factors Associated with the Metabolic Syndrome." *Med Sci Sports Exercise.* 1999; 31:287–293.

17. Gustat JS, Srinivascan J, et al. "Relation of Self-rated Measures of Physical Activity to Multiple Risk Factors of Insulin Resistance Syndrome in Younger Adults: the Bogalusa Heart Study." *J Clin Epidemiology.* 202; 55:997–1006.

18. National Osteoporosis Foundation. "Prevention Exercise for Healthy Bones." Accessed April 2010. www.nof.org/prevention/exercise.htm.

19. Layne J, Nelson M. "The Effects of Progressive Resistance Training on Bone Density: A Review." *Med Sci Sports Exerc.* 1999; 31(1):25–30.

20. American Heart Association. Resistance Exercise in Individuals With and Without Cardiovascular Disease: 2007 Update; A Scientific Statement. Circulation. 2007; 116:572–584.

21. Hoeger W, Hoeger S. *Principles and Labs for Fitness and Wellness: Sixth Edition.* Canada: Wadsworth Thompson: 2002.

22. Wisloff U, Haram P. Brubakk. "Exercise and the Endothelium." In Aird, W.C. *Endothelial Biomedicine.* New York: Cambridge University Press, 2007. 506–511.

23. Siff M, Verkhoshansky, Y. *Supertraining.* Supertraining Institute: 2003.

Chapter 5: Graded Aesthetic Enhancement

1. Perricone, N. *The Perricone Prescription.* New York: HarperCollins, 2002.

2. See Jennie Brand-Miller, M.D., et al. *The New Glucose Revolution,* 3rd edition (Cambridge, MA: Da Capo Press, 2007), for the most comprehensive list of glycemic foods.

3. Goldstein, A.L., J.A. Hooper, R.S. Schulof, et al. "Thymosin and the Immunopathology of Aging." *Fed Proc* 339 (1974): 2053–2056.

4. Fries, J. *Aging Well.* New York: Addison Wesley, 1989.

5. Ibid.

6. Ibid.

7. Perricone, N. *The Perricone Prescription.* New York: HarperCollins, 2002.

8. Kane, M. *The Botox Book.* New York: St. Martin's Press, 2002.

Chapter 6: Restore Bio-Identical Hormones

1. Anderson, A. "The Effects of Exogenous Testosterone on Sexuality and Mood of Normal Men." *J Clin Endocrinol Metabol* 75b (1992): 1503–1507.

2. Rudman, D. "Effects of Growth Hormone Replacement in Men." *N Engl J Med* 323:1 (1990): 1–6.

3. Pierpaoli, W. *Melatonin Miracle.* New York: Simon and Schuster, 1995.

4. Regelson, W. *Super Hormone Promise.* New York: Simon and Schuster, 1996.

5. Rozencwaig, R. *Melatonin and Aging Sourcebook.* Prescott, AZ: Hohm Press, 1997.

6. Pierpaoli, W. *The Melatonin Miracle.* New York: Simon and Schuster, 1995.

7. Barnes, B. *Hypothyroidism: The Unsuspected Illness.* New York: Harper, 1976.

8. Regelson, W., R. Loria, M. Kalimi. "Hormonal Intervention: 'Buffer Hormones' or 'State Dependency.' The Role of Dehydroepiandrosterone (DHEA), Thyroid Hormone, Estrogen and Hypophysectomy in Aging." *Ann NY Acad Sci* 521 (1988): 260–273.

9. Wilson, J. *Adrenal Fatigue.* Petaluma, CA: SMART Publications, 2006.

10. Simpson, G. *Spa Medicine.* Bergen, NJ: Basic Health, 2004.

11. Nankin, H.R., and J.H. Calkins. "Decreased Bio-available Testosterone in Aging Normal and Impotent Men." *J Clin Endocrinol Metabol* 63:6 (1986): 1418–1420.

12. Lichten, Edward, M.D. www.USDOCTOR.com.

13. Kohler, T.S., J. Kim, K. Feia, et al. "Prevalence of Androgen Deficiency in Men with Erectile Dysfunction." *Urology* 71:4 (2008): 693–697.

Chapter 7: Advanced Supplementation

1. Aird, W. *Endothelial Biomedicine.* New York: Cambridge University Press, 2007.

2. Lipton, B. *The Biology of Belief.* New York: Mountain of Love, Elite Books, 2005.

3. Pischinger, A. *The Extracellular Matrix and Ground Regulation.* Berkeley, CA: North Atlantic, 2007.

4. Carrell, A. Nobel lecture, December 11, 1912. Available online at: http://nobel-prize. org/nobel_prizes/medicine/laureates/1912/carrel-lecture.html.

5. Fairfield, K. "Vitamins for Chronic Disease Prevention in Adults." *JAMA* 287 (June 2002): 3116–3129.

6. Young, G. *The pH Miracle for Weight Loss.* New York: Hachette Book Group, 2006.

7. *J Am Diabetic Assoc* 7:Suppl (1997): 31–41.

8. Young, G. *The pH Miracle for Weight Loss.* New York: Hachette Book Group, 2006.

9. Batmanghelidj, F. *Your Body's Many Cries for Water.* Falls Church, VA: Global Health Solutions, 1994.

10. Cobbald, J. *Viktor Schauberger.* London: Floris Books, 2006.

11. Alexandersson, O. *Living Water.* Dublin: Gateway, 1990.

Chapter 8: Lifelong (Mind-Body) Learning

1. Goleman, D. *Mind, Body, Medicine.* New York: Consumer Reports Books, 1993.

2. Benson, H. *Relaxation Response.* New York: Hearst Books, 1976.

3. Keefer, L. "Relaxation and Bowel Dysfunction." *Behav Res Ther* 40 (2002): 541–546.

4. Foa, E.B., B.O. Rothbaum, D.S. Riggs, et al. "Treatment of Posttraumatic Stress Disorder in Rape Victims: A Comparison between Cognitive-behavioral Procedures and Counseling." *J Consult Clin Psychol* 59:5 (1991): 715–723.

5. Childre, D. *Freeze Frame.* Boulder Creek, CA: Planetary Publications, 1994.

6. Wilber, K. *Integral Spirituality.* Boston: Integral Books, 2006.

7. Smith, P. *Killing the Spirit.* New York: Penguin Books, 1990.

8. Snell, B. *The Discovery of the Mind.* Mineola, NY: Dover Publications, 1982.

9. Turner, F. *Beyond Geography.* Piscataway, NJ: Rutgers University Press, 1983.

10. Eccles, J. *Wonder of Being Human.* Boston: Shambhala, 1985.

11. Dunne, B. "Experiments in Remote Human/Machine Interaction." *J Sci Exploration* 6 (1992): 311–332.

12. Targ, R. "Remote Viewing at Stanford Research Institute." *J Sci Exploration* 10:1 (1996): 77–88.

13. Dossey, L. *Healing Words.* San Francisco: Harper, 1993.

Index

About the Author

Graham Simpson, M.D., graduated from the University of the Witwatersrand Medical School in Johannesburg, South Africa, and is board certified in Internal Medicine and Emergency Medicine. Dr. Simpson is a founding member of the American Holistic Medical Association (AHMA) and is also a licensed homeopath. He is the co-author of *Spa Medicine* (Basic Health, 2004) and has taught as an assistant professor of medicine at the University of Nevada, Reno. Dr. Simpson is the medical director of the Ageless Zone Medical Spa in Reno. He is also a consultant for Cenegentics Medical Institute and currently serves as CEO of Eternity Medicine Institute.